THE EVERYTHING.
GUIDE TO
MEDITATION FOR
HEALTHY LIVING

Dear Reader,

You have chosen to make meditation a part of your daily life, which is perhaps one of the best choices you could make for your own personal well-being. The techniques in this book will provide some guidance along the journey, and you will also learn how changes in your body enable successful meditation.

The two of us have journeyed through many forms of meditation over the years, and we hope that some of our experience and learning will help you to find a satisfactory path. Ravi has introduced techniques of meditation to his patients to reduce anxiety and promote healing, and David has taught meditation to his students as part of his mission to reconnect people with animals and nature.

The benefits of meditation can be empirically demonstrated. Meditation lowers blood pressure and cholesterol, improves concentration and memory, and reduces anxiety and depression.

We can all tap into the everyday miracle of meditation by simply setting aside a few minutes each day to foster peace and tranquility. May you find release from the concerns of everyday life and a renewed mind and body as you implement the teachings in this volume and work through the guided sessions on the enclosed CD.

David Dillard-Wright
Ravinder Jerath

Welcome to the EVERYTHING® Series!

These handy, accessible books give you all you need to tackle a difficult project, gain a new hobby, comprehend a fascinating topic, prepare for an exam, or even brush up on something you learned back in school but have since forgotten.

You can choose to read an *Everything®* book from cover to cover or just pick out the information you want from our four useful boxes: e-questions, e-facts, e-alerts, and e-ssentials.

We give you everything you need to know on the subject, but throw in a lot of fun stuff along the way, too.

We now have more than 400 *Everything®* books in print, spanning such wide-ranging categories as weddings, pregnancy, cooking, music instruction, foreign language, crafts, pets, New Age, and so much more. When you're done reading them all, you can finally say you know *Everything®*!

QUESTION

Answers to
common questions

FACT

Important snippets
of information

ALERT

Urgent
warnings

ESSENTIAL

Quick
handy tips

PUBLISHER Karen Cooper

DIRECTOR OF ACQUISITIONS AND INNOVATION Paula Munier

MANAGING EDITOR, EVERYTHING® SERIES Lisa Laing

COPY CHIEF Casey Ebert

ASSISTANT PRODUCTION EDITOR Jacob Erickson

ACQUISITIONS EDITOR Lisa Laing

DEVELOPMENT EDITOR Katrina Schroeder

EDITORIAL ASSISTANT Ross Weisman

EVERYTHING® SERIES COVER DESIGNER Erin Alexander

LAYOUT DESIGNERS Colleen Cunningham, Elisabeth Lariviere, Ashley Vierra, Denise Wallace

Visit the entire Everything® series at *www.everything.com*

THE
EVERYTHING®
GUIDE TO MEDITATION FOR HEALTHY LIVING

Reduce stress, improve health,
and increase longevity

David B. Dillard-Wright, PhD and Ravinder Jerath, MD

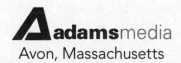

Aadamsmedia
Avon, Massachusetts

For Oscar

An Everything® Series Book.
Everything® and everything.com® are registered trademarks of F+W Media, Inc.

Published by Adams Media, a division of F+W Media, Inc.
57 Littlefield Street, Avon, MA 02322 U.S.A.
www.adamsmedia.com

ISBN 10: 1-4405-1088-1
ISBN 13: 978-1-4405-1088-5
eISBN 10: 1-4405-1151-9
eISBN 13: 978-1-4405-1151-6

Printed in the United States of America.

10 9 8 7 6 5 4 3 2 1

Library of Congress Cataloging-in-Publication Data
Dillard-Wright, David B.
The everything guide to meditation for healthy living / David B. Dillard-Wright and Ravinder Jerath.
    p. cm. — (Everything)
ISBN-13: 978-1-4405-1088-5
ISBN-10: 1-4405-1088-1
ISBN-13: 978-1-4405-1151-6 (ebk)
ISBN-10: 1-4405-1151-9 (ebk)
1. Meditation I. Jerath, Ravinder. II. Title.
BL627.D55 2010
204'.35—dc22
          2010038805

This book is available at quantity discounts for bulk purchases.
For information, please call 1-800-289-0963.

Contents

Acknowledgments

The authors would like to thank Greenbough House of Prayer, The Monastery of the Holy Spirit, The Monastery of the Glorious Ascension, Himalayan Academy, International Sivananda Yoga Vedanta Centers, Dharma Pravartaka Acharya, Vamadeva Shastri, the University of South Carolina Aiken, and the Augusta Hindu Temple Society for their support and inspiration.

The Top 10 Reasons to Begin Meditating Today

1. Because you are envious of the happy expression on your dog's face.

2. Because life doesn't come with a reset button.

3. Because you want to want to get out of bed in the morning.

4. Because coffee isn't cutting it anymore.

5. Because they don't make industrial-strength vitamins.

6. Because you have always secretly wanted a nature-sounds CD.

7. Because your boss will not, apparently, be hiring an assistant for you.

8. Because you owe it to yourself.

9. Because today is the first day of the rest of your life.

10. Because you're human.

Introduction

Meditation is recommended as one of the basic tools for just about every path to self-improvement or spiritual practice. Meditations in churches, temples, and mosques unite people in mind and spirit. In secular life, meditations for group therapy, celebrations, and memorials give us moments to reflect and remember important things. And when a vital message is passed on to us, we may be asked to meditate on it. Meditation is more a part of our lives than we realize.

Meditation is supposed to quiet you, to focus your mind on just one thing. While it's possible for most of us to accomplish this focus, it usually doesn't last long. The business of living must be tended to, so we go on to other things. Work, home, and social life are important, and meditation appears to have little to do with them. Who has the time to do nothing?

Actually, the practice of meditation should be at the core of our life. It's the basic tool that allows every act to have meaning and richness. Meditation doesn't have to be a separate, "special" event that takes us away from our responsibilities or leisure. It can be an ongoing process that is part of everything that we do.

If you've had experience with meditation, maybe you took it for granted as time went by. You may have started with the basics and became discouraged when you didn't see the results you expected. So you went off to learn other things that seemed more interesting. Or, maybe you never really got the chance to learn to meditate; you just imitated those around you by being quiet and respectful.

If meditation is an idea you want to explore, what is the best way to go about it? And if you occasionally meditate, how can you develop and grow with it?

There are many approaches to meditation. Some may appear to be simple and practical; others may seem otherworldly and impractical. You may find books on styles or schools of meditation that present words and concepts that are way over your head. Or you may have looked into classes that turn out to be too religious, or not spiritual enough.

To find the meditation style that best suits you, it's fair to look at what each style offers and decide what features are suitable—for you. You'll have an opportunity to do that with this book. You'll learn that it's not necessary to limit yourself to one meditation style. We live in an age when nearly all of the meditation traditions have come out of cultural isolation to offer a variety of paths for self-discovery. By incorporating what reflects your unique nature, whether it is two or three styles, or a dozen, you will be able to design a meditation practice that reflects all that you are.

As you begin, you will discover the keys that open the door to your potential as a human being. You'll enter a vast and beautiful dimension that all who have lived before you discovered in some way through life. In this place you'll find ways of meeting challenges and coping with problems. You'll also find new ways to engage your life with experience that teaches, heals, and enhances everything around you. It will take some work, but it is a labor of love you deserve to give yourself.

If discovering greater meaning and purpose in life isn't reason enough to begin a meditation practice, the physical benefits should be. Over the past few decades, evidence has been mounting which suggests that meditation helps to reduce the harmful effects of stressful lifestyles. Want to have more energy? Reduce the risk of a heart attack? Control depression and anxiety? Oftentimes, our first response to such problems is to reach for a pill bottle, but perhaps more ancient ways of combating them should be employed alongside modern Western medicine. Perhaps people living thousands of years ago had some wisdom about life that we have lost with our fast paced, technology-driven societies. And yet, at the same time, our technology and science help us to understand ancient practices better, to find empirical explanations for how and why they work. In this book, you will find a mixture of ancient practices and scientific explanation, and you will see how differing schools of thought agree that meditation really does promote healthy living.

CHAPTER 1

What Is Meditation?

Meditation is often recommended as a remedy for the ills of modern living: stress, anxiety, depression, and poor health. It is praised for its healing benefits and positive influence on personal well-being and relationships. "I'll meditate on that" is an everyday response to a wide number of social, business, and personal situations that call for reflection.

To Meditate or Not to Meditate

What, exactly, is meditation? Briefly described, meditation is the stilling of all your conscious faculties in order to be present in the moment. But why is this so important?

How Others See Meditation

Even though meditation is beneficial, those who meditate are sometimes portrayed as sitting in painful positions for hours, just waiting for something good to happen. Some people may think that people who meditate are hiding from reality.

FACT

The great religious and philosophical traditions all agree that the dimensions of body, mind, and spirit coexist for a reason. Certain practices have arisen out of this view, and meditation is one of them. It's known in many forms—such as prayer, silence, and stillness—but it is universally recognized and employed. Meditation is a tool for coordinating and harmonizing the body, mind, and spirit in our lives.

At the same time, those who meditate regularly and conscientiously appear to be serene about things that exasperate the rest of us. And they seem to have so much vitality! But we often hold back from trying to understand more about the subject.

What Meditation Does for You

Perhaps you believe that we are composed of more than flesh and bone, that everyone possesses a mind and spirit as well. This is neither a spiritual nor a metaphysical view.

But even if we accept this view of human nature, understanding the relationships between body, mind, and spirit has posed an age-old challenge. Which dimension has priority in everyday life? For example, do the needs of the body dictate the requirements of the mind: does eating take precedence over learning?

Likewise, questions of the spirit pose greater quandaries. After all, the realm of spirit is intangible, so many disciplines lay claim to it. Religion, philosophy, and science each vie for our allegiance by providing characteristic labels for the needs of the spirit. For example, religious belief categorizes the world of spirit according to theological doctrines that stem from past traditions and cultural beliefs. Philosophy places the realm of spirit beyond cognitive learning. As such, spiritual existence is a proposition rather than a reality. But if spirit does exist, it can only be known by studying human nature and reason. And in science, physicists allude to a spiritual dimension as the cosmology of our universe. It is viewed as conscious matter or energy, depending on the scientific approach employed.

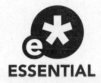

ESSENTIAL

Who needs meditation? Everyone can benefit from meditation. Students need meditation to help them memorize information and relax before exams. Office workers need meditation to prevent preoccupation with detail and to help see the big picture. People who work at home need meditation to avoid feelings of isolation while coping with the day's demands.

Why People Meditate

People meditate for many different reasons. You may want to learn about meditation from simple curiosity or because of a particular need. Looking at some of the following conditions that influence practitioners of meditation may help you discover why you seek the way to this practice.

- **Anger:** A condition of continual upset that makes it impossible to maintain calm even away from the people and things that are provocative. Meditation provides calming time, an opportunity to see those people and things differently.
- **Curiosity:** The need to know all personal dimensions, to have the courage to explore them, and to experience the reality of true self. This is a noble goal and the key motive for practicing meditation.

- **Depression:** A state in which life seems without purpose, although there is clearly more to it than present experiences. Meditation can help you find the innate serenity you possess.
- **Fear:** Everything you do takes more work because you're not sure whether something will sabotage your efforts. Meditation helps find the places in the mind and heart that are vulnerable and heals them.
- **Pain:** A condition of sadness, perhaps from a loss or a major disappointment. Meditation can bring acceptance of the situation and discovery of inner strengths to anticipate new, rewarding experiences.
- **Stress:** You are frazzled from the routine of your life and the demands it makes on you. Meditation can help you cope and even provide the means to change your situation.

What Meditation Is and Isn't

Many people have heard of meditation, but few really know what it is. As a result, there are many widespread misconceptions.

ALERT

Meditation is not the final goal. As a means toward the harmonizing of our different dimensions, meditation leads to innumerable benefits. Each tradition and meditation discipline emphasizes one or several of those benefits. It is up to you to determine the goal and the traditional approach to meet that goal.

Misconceptions about Meditation

When considering meditation, some erroneous images may come to mind. For example, there is the ascetic sitting cross-legged on a mountaintop far from the realities of everyday life. With eyes closed, perfect posture, and an immobile expression, the meditator appears to be in another world, above and beyond the demands that the rest of us are dealing with on a daily basis. This image seems neither possible to emulate, nor a worthwhile goal.

Seasoned meditators will quickly and knowingly dismiss these impressions. Meditation, they say, is a natural condition and requires no special separation from daily life. And you do not have to give up your creature comforts. In fact, meditation allows you to appreciate and understand their presence in your life.

In addition, although perfect posture and immobility are skills that can be learned through meditation, they are not the purpose of practice. Physical conditioning does play a fundamental role in meditation, but you don't have to stand on your head or contort your body to achieve balance or harmony. Natural postures, movements, and breathing are all that you need to start a meditation practice. You may quickly learn, however, that what you have been doing for some time is not natural after all. So relearning breathing and practicing natural sitting and stance may become part of your learning program.

People also assume that the meditative state is somehow removed from reality, or that we have to absent ourselves from everyday existence to be truly meditative. Nothing could be further from the truth. Because, once again, traditional meditation systems point out that the stresses and demands on our attention remove us from the true reality, which is the meditative state.

Well, what if your outer life is so pressing that you need an escape once in a while? This is a legitimate concern that everyone will have eventually. In this instance, meditation is not an escape. It is a way that we can understand why life is difficult at times and adjust our response accordingly. This may sound like a tall order, but most meditation traditions emphasize that we can understand the true nature of reality through meditation. This enables us not only to cope with it, but actually to work through challenging times and see the value they offer. At the same time, we can find that escape by recognizing as illusions our everyday "pressing matters."

Meditation by Any Other Name

Meditation strikes many as a religious practice, one that requires strict adherence to a creed that is unfamiliar and foreign to our established beliefs. Again, this assumption is far from the truth: Meditation is an innate part of every spiritual tradition, although it may not be named as such. Prayer, contemplation, silence, and ceremony are all meditative acts. They can be found in every religion, ancient and modern, and they are vital to strengthening faith and belief. Some meditation techniques are identical in different religious practices, even though they are called by different names. For example, *asana* (from Sanskrit, meaning "to sit") is a basic meditation practice in Yoga (meaning "yoke" or "union," the psycho-physical techniques deriving from Hinduism), while in the Buddhist practice of Zen, *zazen* (from Japanese, meaning "sitting") is the same approach.

ESSENTIAL

Meditation is as old as human existence. It has been practiced religiously and philosophically. Every spiritual movement, no matter how great or small, has an established meditative tradition. Some secular techniques have also developed that offer the same valuable results. These include many forms of art, dance, music, ceremony, martial arts disciplines, and communing with nature.

Similarly, the Native American will "follow the spirit quest" while a Middle Eastern Sufi spins in a wondrous dance of ecstasy to know oneness with the Creator. What these activities have in common is the use of a particular meditative approach to experience spirituality. Meditation is the tool; spirituality is the goal. Meditation is the journey to discover the place where the heart lives, where you can meet your true self. As one teacher said, "There's no avoiding spirit in meditation, you will encounter it."

For the practitioner who is not religious, meditation dispenses with the requirement of belief, because it is based in self-awareness and personal experience. These are valuable approaches to developing a meditation practice that is truly individual and nondenominational.

Meditating Without Knowing It

What is it like to meditate? This inside joke in the consciousness movement provides a clever answer: Meditation is not what you think. Did you know that you often enter a meditative state under everyday circumstances without knowing it? The natural trend toward self-awareness can often come from performing simple, methodical tasks that free the mind from concentrated thought. Such tasks often disengage feelings, which can distract your attention. For example:

- **Engaging in challenging sports:** Athletes frequently speak of the mental freedom that is attained when the body is so completely involved in meeting a challenge, such as running a long distance or climbing a steep incline.
- **Nursing a baby:** Mothers know that the serenity that accompanies breastfeeding enhances the bonding process with the infant and also brings a deep perception of the life force itself.
- **Performing strenuous physical work:** Laborers know that the rigor of a physical task, such as carrying heavy loads with great care, can bring uncommon mind-body awareness.
- **Washing dishes:** Performing such a familiar task often frees the mind to become aware of itself.

In these instances it is the realization—without thought or feeling—that you are participating in the moment that brings you into the state of meditation.

What You Will Gain Through Meditation

Meditation is often recommended as a remedy for many of the problems we face in our modern age. We are beginning to learn that stress, isolation, fear, and illness can be alleviated in substantial ways by meditation. Many professionals acknowledge this benefit and incorporate meditation as an essential component of good health.

The Effects of Meditation on Your Physical Health

In the early 1990s, cardiovascular physician Dean Ornish, from the University of Texas Medical Center, set the conventional medical world on end when he offered documented proof that heart disease can be halted and even reversed by changing lifestyle. According to his research and a unique program he developed for patients, meditation figured prominently in this breakthrough. Dr. Ornish designed a regimen that combined diet, exercise, and the regular practice of meditation to assist in healing heart patients in his program. The results far exceeded expectations. He reported dramatic recoveries from cardiovascular disease—82 percent in one year. Dr. Ornish, a longtime follower of the Yoga teacher Swami Satchidananda, applied his years as a meditator to show the way toward restored health for the thousands of heart patients who followed.

In the 1970s, studies on the effects of transcendental meditation conducted at the Los Angeles Center for the Health Sciences showed that heart rate, blood pressure, and some endocrine secretions are altered to healthful levels in the meditative state. This effect on so-called involuntary physiological functions is good reason to include meditation in the repertoire of preventive medicine.

In the last decade, researchers have used magnetic resonance imaging (MRI) to map the effects of meditation on the brain and electroencephalography (EEG) to measure brain waves. At the same time, larger studies have been conducted with groups of actual patients to determine the effects of meditation on health. The results suggest that meditation has an effect on the body that is similar to deep sleep, enabling the body to reset its systems and repair ongoing damage. While more work still needs to be done, evidence that meditation has numerous health benefits is irrefutable.

FACT

Some public schools in San Francisco have begun incorporating meditation in their physical education classes. Initially offered to students as Kiddie Yoga, this option was intended to help strengthen the body. But teachers have also noted that the meditative breathing exercises also help students focus on academic tasks. The students have reported that they are more relaxed before tests, and even look forward to them.

Endorphins, the natural brain chemicals that produce a state of well-being, are a necessary component in maintaining mental and emotional balance. These chemicals not only promote good feelings, they assist in boosting the immune system. Meditation has been found to play a significant part in promoting the flow of endorphins, and this has great value in addressing the problems of anxiety and panic disorders.

The Effects of Meditation on the Mind

The practice of meditation requires a faculty we depend on every moment of every day—the mind. But the literature of meditation, from pragmatic approaches to psychospiritual teachings, is loaded with references to the difficulties the mind poses. We may discover that in fact, the mind obstructs the awareness we seek. Thinking, analyzing, and worrying are all examples of this obstruction. As a result, some sources emphasize techniques for controlling, relaxing, and focusing the mind. Some of these techniques supposedly take months and years to master and may even require a teacher to monitor progress.

QUOTE

"To become different from what we are, we must have some awareness of what we are."

—Bruce Lee, *Tao of Jeet Kune Do*

However, the many traditions of meditation demonstrate that we do not need to impose such constraints on our minds. The mind can be a helpful vehicle that transports us to new states of being. We can discover the wonderful facets that our minds possess and use those functions to develop truly enhanced mental skills. But to do this, we must first learn how to exercise the mind in beneficial ways—and that is one of the vital reasons meditation is so important.

The Mental Dimension

Psychologists are quick to point out that the mental faculty consists of several components or levels. The different meditation paths support this view as well. Understanding these components is an important step in forging a meditation practice, because we will encounter these levels in different ways as we learn meditation exercises and techniques.

The Waking Conscious

The conscious mind is what we are most familiar with. It is our immediate involvement with the present and encompasses the functions of our senses. Sight, hearing, touch, taste, and scent involve our attention and evoke responses that we may or may not manage according to our will. The waking conscious constantly brings information and challenges to our attention. Associating, recognizing, analyzing, and comparing are all functions of this level.

FACT

Consciousness is the active awareness of your mental and physical state, with the ability to modify these states. Brain-injured individuals can sometimes be fully conscious but unable to communicate or modify their physical state even though their mental state is active and aware.

The waking conscious is a fundamental and necessary component of existence. No meditation practice will exclude that; so don't worry about "losing consciousness" or entering a trance or deep state of hypnosis. In fact, meditation depends on a well-developed waking conscious mind. Many meditation exercises will assist in making this possible.

The Unconscious

The unconscious is sometimes called the subconscious, what is below or beneath consciousness. It is a realm to which psychology and religion have given great attention, and for good reason. The unconscious stores everything that the waking conscious delegates to the back burner, so to speak. The unconscious also possesses memories, symbols, feelings, and thoughts that are not pertinent to our immediate needs.

An example of the power of the unconscious is the activity of dreams. We certainly don't dictate to the unconscious what we will dream, when, where, or the topic. The unconscious produces activity and information according to its own agenda, which is certainly our agenda but not necessarily our choice. So we are, in a sense, subject to the currents of the unconscious mind.

Meditation is a proven way to reach and understand the unconscious mind. In fact, some preliminary meditation experiences may evoke images and insights into the unconscious that are surprising or unsettling. But the more that meditation is practiced, the more familiar this territory becomes. The unconscious mind can yield solutions to pressing problems and awaken strengths we never knew we had. In addition, those "involuntary" levels, such as physiological states and emotional expression, are found in the unconscious. It becomes possible to communicate with those levels through meditation.

The Superconscious

Different traditions view the superconscious in different ways and call it by different names, but the premise is basically the same: the intangible, spiritual nature of human existence. It is the self in Jungian psychology, the soul of Christianity, the divine body of several mystical traditions, the *atman* in Yoga philosophy, and the Buddha nature in Buddhism.

FACT

Aristotle thought the human heart was the seat of consciousness. Plato believed it was within the brain. Descartes described the pineal gland in the brain as the control center of the body and mind. Eventually two schools of thought were established to explain the brain-mind connection: dualism (which teaches that the mind is independent of the brain) and monism (which teaches that the mind is located within the brain).

Is knowledge of the superconscious possible? According to most meditation systems, it certainly is. In fact, the goal of many schools is not only to discover this dimension but to integrate it with the mind and body to achieve the full realization of our potential as human beings. The superconscious is also seen as a dimension in which we can cultivate advanced powers such as healing, hypersense, and rejuvenation. There are many examples of this potential: the physical prowess of yogis and practitioners of the martial arts, the longevity of meditation masters, and the marvelous calm and serenity achieved by those who embrace deep prayer and devoted work.

Is this potential accessible by ordinary people? According to both secular and religious meditation traditions, it is the inevitable result of consistent and dedicated practice.

All the traditional meditation systems agree that reaching the superconscious is a gradual process that requires constant practice and dedicated work. That is why meditation is called a practice, because it is a continuous process of unfolding our skill to reach beyond our ordinary state of awareness.

How to Balance the Body and the Spirit

If, according to the philosophy of monism, the mind operates within the confines of the physical brain, then the physical realm is something that cannot be circumvented in meditation. What can be done to still the body from its incessant thirsts and hungers, and balance the needs of the flesh with the spirit? This dilemma has been faced by the human race from time immemorial. And many solutions have been devised, employed, discarded, or passed on in the process.

Suffering the Body

Some schools of meditation suffer the body while focusing on higher realities, making do with material existence. Certain disciplines and methods may be imposed that involve trained observation of the physical functions, so the practitioner can see how he breathes, for instance, and how the senses react to outside stimulation. By gradually understanding how the body works, its functions can be calmed and stilled. Detachment from the physical is emphasized in this approach, and the practitioner is able, for example, to sit on beds of nails or walk over burning coals without injury.

Celebrating the Body

Other meditation schools may work in the opposite direction—fully employing the physical senses to know certain realities in the mental, emotional, and psychic ("of the psyche") realms. Here, the rhythms of the body and nature are completely but consciously engaged in their natural course, which allows the practitioner to perceive the underlying forces that interact with existence.

Both approaches are common to a number of meditation practices, but they are extreme and not the "middle way" (as Buddhist philosophy expresses it). In the beginning, some of the techniques in the classical meditation systems—such as controlling heart rate or detecting the presence of wild animals in the environs—are quite useful to learn and understand. These techniques convey the powers of self-control and awareness, but they are not the aim of the meditation journey. Rather, the initial goal is to cultivate a curiosity about yourself and eventually come to understand as many of your dimensions as possible—body, mind, and even the soul.

FACT

In the 1960s, Harvard psychology professor Richard Alpert left the academic world to become a prime mover in the nascent consciousness movement. Alpert studied meditation with Indian teachers and emerged as Baba Ram Dass, a teacher of Eastern traditions who urged seekers of the inner life to "be here now," a dictum that titled his 1971 book on practical mysticism.

The Language of Consciousness

While certain words have established meanings, in the context of meditation practice they can take on other meanings as well. Words represent conscious powers that we can exercise in meditation.

- **Awareness:** Using the physical senses to enhance our perception of the present involves the faculties of hearing, seeing, body sensation, and breath.
- **Contemplation:** Using all your faculties (the senses of sight, sound, touch, smell, taste, and conscious attention) to learn as much as possible about one idea or image allows all of our senses to become consciously involved in an experience.
- **Focus:** Placing attention on a single idea or image retrains it to that singularity when attention moves away from it.
- **Visualization:** Bringing to mind an object or scene that assists in fulfilling a specific purpose stimulates the subtle powers of the body to follow this course.

CHAPTER 2

The Physiology of Meditation

A variety of scientific studies over several decades have established that meditation lowers blood pressure and heart rate and even affects cholesterol levels. Meditation has also been used to treat anxiety and depression and a wide variety of other psychological and physiological disorders. Indeed, the health benefits of meditation lead many to begin a meditation practice in the first place. There are a multitude of changes that take place in the body as a result of conscious control of breathing and thoughts. Knowing about the physiology of mind and meditation will give you a deeper appreciation for what happens each time you take a breath.

The Dynamic Model of Consciousness

Common sense says that the brain commands and controls the rest of the body, like a puppet master controls the strings of a puppet, or like a drill sergeant barks orders at cadets. The command-and-control idea of the brain has a certain amount of truth to it, but the reality is actually much more cooperative than this image allows. "Mind," which actually includes more than just the brain, describes the ways that the body's many systems interact with the brain and the environment to produce experiences.

The relationship between brain and body is by no means a one-way process: not only does the brain dictate to the body, but the body also dictates to the brain. It might be better to think of the body's many systems and its immediate surroundings as a dense web of relationships. These relationships are nonlocal and dispersed, meaning that a change in any one area can affect the whole body. Even below the system level, cellular processes also have a certain logic and are affected by events taking place throughout the body. All of this means that any bodily process, whether healthful or harmful, can be altered by manipulating the body's electrical and informational processes through meditation.

FACT

The body contains around 100 billion neurons, capable of sending impulses at the rate of up to 400 feet per second.

Think of your "mind" as a triangle consisting of the brain, your body, and the surrounding environment. Each of the three points in this system has a complex structure of its own. The brain has numerous processing centers. Neural elements extend downward into the heart and lungs, and, through the spinal column, reach every part of the body. Then there are the other processes taking place in the body: respiration, circulation, and digestion, for example, as well as endocrine and renal functioning. The organs, systems, and cells of the body execute trillions of functions every second, and the wondrous part of it all is that the vast majority of it happens without any conscious effort on the part of the rational mind.

That said, the thoughts that pass through your head and the emotions associated with those thoughts *do* matter and can affect all of these unseen processes to a profound degree. The quality of the environment certainly also affects consciousness and health. For example, depriving a person of a suitable and stimulating environment will impair social and cognitive development, just as a very rich environment will produce a rich intellectual and emotional life.

Some things lie outside of your control. You can't alter your DNA, for example (at least not yet), and you have to put up with a certain amount of toxicity and stress as part of our modern, industrialized consumer lifestyles. You may even have persistent (though not inevitable) features of your personality that can be very difficult to overcome. Anger, depression, and anxiety have become invisible plagues in society, affecting almost every aspect of our common life. Given the state of the world today with the steady stream of bad news about the environment, economics, and politics, it might be tempting to just go along with the flow and forget about living a healthy, centered lifestyle.

Fortunately, meditation and deep, slow breathing (pranayama) can balance the triangle of body, brain, and environment, returning our experience of the world to a more neutral, peaceful state. The ancient wisdom of the world's philosophies and religions as expressed in prayer and meditation can now be scientifically verified and understood physiologically. Prayer and breathing are proving to be a formidable force that can create natural sunshine within while thunderstorms and hail may be raging outside. Neurology, biology, medicine, and a whole variety of subfields describe the ways in which meditation works to an amazing degree of specificity, but here we simply want to capture the general outlines.

Thinking Through Breathing

When you inhale, air enters your bronchial passageways and travels into tiny sacs called alveoli. Here, the blood exchanges gases with the air in the lungs: the more oxygenated air replaces the exhaled carbon dioxide. This is all made possible by the mixture of gases available in the atmosphere on the earth, which, with the exception of very high altitudes and artificial, undersea breathing, has just the right amount of oxygen to allow the body's cells to break down food and convert it to energy. Too much oxygen damages cells just as much as having too little oxygen. According to some theories, oxygen free radicals, released in the process of nourishing cells, actually cause aging, and yet an absence of oxygen leads to brain damage in minutes. Optimum oxygen consumption minimizes damage to cells while giving them what they need to carry out their functions.

Deep Breathing and Oxygen Intake

Deep, slow breathing actually causes the cells to consume less, not more oxygen, reducing the amount of stress on the body. This kind of breathing has the same effect as small, regular meals have on your calorie intake. If you starve yourself during a busy day or because of some emotional upset, the usual outcome is a binge afterward. A skipped lunch may become a late afternoon break for candy and soda. When the body experiences gaps in regular eating, it compensates by lowering metabolism to conserve energy. In the same way, deep slow breathing produces increased oxygenation, which means that a lower blood flow can carry the same amount of oxygen. The heart doesn't have to work as hard to supply the body with oxygen, which leads to lowered blood pressure and a lower heart rate. The effect on your heart is similar to the effect of aerobic exercise.

QUOTE

> Just as rain pierces a poorly roofed house,
> so passion pierces an uncultivated mind.
> Just as rain cannot pierce a well-roofed house,
> so passion cannot pierce a well-cultivated mind.
>
> —The Buddha

Breathing deeply is like saying to the circulatory system, "Look, everything is okay. Just relax. I've got you covered." Some yogis (practitioners of Yoga) believe that short breaths lead to a short lifespan, while long breaths lead to a long lifespan. While it would be difficult to quantify the effects of deep breathing over a lifetime of practice, evidence suggests that deliberate, regular practice will relieve high blood pressure and cardiovascular disease. It does not seem like too big of a leap to conclude that the practice of deep breathing could also help prevent these conditions.

Diffusing Fight-or-Flight

The lung-heart interconnection is one way in which deep breathing and meditation affects health, but it is not the only way. Neural elements in the lungs called stretch receptors also play a role in the relaxing effects of meditation. Under stress, the brain sends signals to the heart and lungs to work harder. This is part of the body's "fight-or-flight" response to a perceived threat. Rapid breathing and heartbeat increases your ability to deal with a threat, like a predator, but it does little good in contemporary life, especially when the stress becomes a daily reality. Under stress, your body works very hard just to maintain functioning, and few resources are left to maintain a clear mental state. A corporate executive may feel highly productive when working in an adrenaline-driven, fast-paced fashion, but mentally she is not functioning at peak capacity.

Fight-or-flight may be the proper response in a crisis, but it is not a good way to function regularly. Such a state leads to clouded, short-term thinking, and is similar to functioning under sleep deprivation or severe exhaustion. When the lungs are more fully inflated, however, the stretch receptors send a message to the brain that slows down and eventually stops the fight-or-flight response. The brain follows the lungs' cues and stops producing the high levels of cortisol and adrenaline also associated with fight-or-flight. These chemicals are capable of producing rapid bursts of energy, but lead to lower levels of energy when overused. Meditation gets the brain and the body out of the "emergency" mode and restores normal, baseline functioning, so that resources are not being wasted in order to counter nonexistent emergencies.

Combining Deep, Slow Breathing with Positive Visualization

Beyond the deep breathing aspect of meditation, the thinking process also plays an important role. You may have noticed how a single negative thought leads to a chain of other negative thoughts. You stub your toe getting out of bed, and, after some other choice phrases, say to yourself, "this just isn't my day." The negative aspects of the morning are then multiplied: the commute seems more annoying than usual, as do the e-mails in your inbox. By mid-morning you feel like screaming and you have a headache, and it only gets worse from there.

In this case, the brain and the body have entered into a negative feedback loop. Negative thoughts induce a negative emotional state, which has a physiological response. Emotional turmoil triggers the fight-or-flight response, and, after the rush subsides, you are left feeling wasted, in a state that feels much like a hangover. You might have feelings of sadness and inadequacy, along with physical pain and a general sense of lethargy. A coffee break helps but doesn't really get rid of the problem, and the cycle begins all over again. This fairly typical response to the problems of life is a boom and bust cycle of overdrive and lull. A person living like this will have a sense that the day is too short to get everything done, because half the time has been spent in a stress-induced coma. This is an unhappy state when one does not have time to smell the roses or appreciate the sky during sunset.

QUOTE

"If we pause and breathe in and out, then we can have the experience of timeless presence, of the inexpressible wisdom and goodness of our own minds. We can look at the world with fresh eyes and hear things with fresh ears."

— Pema Chödrön

Some fortunate souls have the opposite response in which a positive thought triggers another positive thought, and so on. Philosopher and psychologist William James called these naturally optimistic types "healthy minded." Nothing seems to upset them, and they sail through life with a cheerful smile. Sometimes such an attitude comes from a deep wisdom, but it can also be a form of camouflage that hides a variety of mental states that are close to those of their more gloomy counterparts. Keeping "on the sunny side" is very hard to achieve for most people, because the universe is a chaotic place, and we are bound to experience setbacks and disappointments. Sheer mental discipline alone is not likely to work as a means of maintaining a good disposition, because we can never be fully prepared for everything that comes our way.

Meditation can help with the process of negotiating life's woes, not by making everything peachy keen, but by pausing the downward cycle of negative thoughts and feelings. The purpose of visualization and mantra practice is to put a placeholder before consciousness that interrupts the flow of oppressive, dark thoughts and emotions. Rather than fighting the negative thoughts and emotions, mantra and visualization *replace* negative thoughts and emotions. The body will begin to believe in the visualization and will stop responding as though the world were falling apart. Positive visualizations achieve some of the same effects as deep, slow breathing. When combined, these two techniques can be a powerful antidote to stress-induced disorders.

Physicians and researchers have long known that illness has a psychosomatic component, and that the "placebo effect" can generate seemingly miraculous cures. What has been less emphasized is the fact that *every* illness has psychosomatic components that can trigger the ailment or prolong it into a chronic state. Anxiety, insomnia, depression, anger disorder, hypertension, and heart disease are just a few of the conditions that can be improved with meditation. The psychosomatic components of these conditions should not be dismissed as beside the point of real therapy or treatment, because, for some conditions, meditation can be as effective as any drug or therapy if used consistently. Our emotional and mental lives are just as much a part of ourselves as our organs, so it makes sense to treat the disorder at the root by improving our experiences through meditation.

Managing Pain, Stress, Fear, and Anxiety with Meditation

Everyone has heard stories of executives working hard for thirty or forty years only to drop dead of a heart attack on the day after retirement. The loss of meaning and purpose in life during major transitions creates a kind of negative feedback loop. Because the brain and the body are an interactive system, what happens emotionally affects health in measurable ways. Many large companies have started extending mental health benefits to their employees, because psychiatric and psychological care can reduce the number of medical claims. Wellness programs similarly create happier and more productive employees. When the mind is functioning well, the body functions well, and vice versa.

Controlling Pain through Meditation

Even pain itself can be altered through mental and social conditioning. The mind and emotions can either magnify or reduce the perception of pain, depending on how a patient chooses to respond to pain. Doctors in a variety of fields prescribe a variety of meditative techniques to reduce pain and anxiety for patients undergoing difficult procedures. Many studies have shown that meditation produces results equal or superior to prescription painkillers. While it would be irresponsible to simply discontinue use of prescribed medications, meditation and breath control, when properly used, can augment the healing effects of medical treatments and minimize their side effects. Meditation also does what no chemical substance will ever be able to do—improve quality of life. Regular meditation gives practitioners more mental space— maneuvering room to solve problems and think creatively—that would not be available to someone functioning in perpetual stress response. It is a passport to freedom of mind and discovery of one's true unlimited potential.

Meditation and Chronic Stress

Living a highly stressful lifestyle without a strategy for dealing with stress leads to a number of conditions. Depression, anxiety, and sleep disorders manifest themselves as early signs of un-processed stress. People with elevated stress levels often complain of a lack of energy, even though they often work long hours. Deeper probing of a hectic work schedule reveals that many of these hours spent at work are unproductive because of a loss of mental clarity, or an inability to concentrate because of other pressing concerns. A workaholic may feel productive, but she is actually under-functioning due to an out-of-control stress response, which produces cloudy short-term judgment. Long-term consequences are even greater. Extended periods of shallow breathing, combined with the increased cortisol and adrenaline (stress hormone) production due to the fight-or-flight response, lead to high blood pressure, heart disease, and possibly diabetes. Often diet and exercise are compromised as a result of a poor coping strategy, compounding the problems further.

By contrast, meditators can stop this downward spiral before it gets out of control. The physiological effects of meditating are similar to exercise in many ways. Meditating, especially when it includes deep, slow breathing, lowers blood pressure and controls the production of stress hormones. The body's systems are recalibrated and begin to work harmoniously again. This is the same kind of tune-up that the body receives in deep sleep. Meditation allows the body's systems to rest and recuperate from the typical overdrive state.

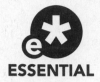

ESSENTIAL

The sympathetic nervous system prepares the body for action by increasing heart rate, constricting the arteries, dilating the pupils, and releasing adrenaline and cortisol (stress hormones). The parasympathetic nervous system returns the body to normal by dilating the arteries, constricting the pupils, slowing the heart rate, and inhibiting the production of stress hormones. Meditation works by stimulating the parasympathetic response.

As a meditator, you will learn to step back and see your thoughts and emotions like the weather—constantly changing but ultimately not very important. You can wean yourself off the roller coaster of the stress response and find a more level state of being, increasing your perceived energy level. This may initially be disconcerting if you have lived with inner turmoil for years or decades. Having a peaceful state of mind may even feel irresponsible, because you have come to think of out-of-control emotions as somehow productive.

Transitioning Away from Fear and Anxiety

Fear and anxiety don't solve problems. You may unconsciously be using powerful emotions as a substitute for constructive action. Meditation takes away the worries, and with them your defenses and excuses. You can see problems and the resources needed to face those problems more clearly. While many exaggerated claims have been made about the potential of meditation to generate worldly success, it can safely be concluded that a sensible program of meditation will produce a more poised and relaxed state of mind that, over time, will lead to a greater quality of life, including greater productivity and quality of work.

Sympathetic and Parasympathetic Balance

To understand how meditation works, you should understand the connections between the sympathetic and parasympathetic nervous systems. When you sleep, your nervous system shifts back and forth between sympathetic-dominant and parasympathetic-dominant states about every one and a half hours. Rapid eye movement (REM) sleep, the state that induces vivid dreaming, is a sympathetic-dominant state. In this part of the sleep cycle, your mind is in a very active mode. Many of the same processes occur in the brain during a dreamed cocktail party as would occur in its "real" counterpart. By contrast, the parasympathetic-dominant state typically is characterized by dreamless sleep, and this is when the rejuvenation of brain and body takes place.

In deep sleep, the rhythm of breathing synchronizes with brain waves. Breathing slows, and so do your brain waves. Meditation, without inducing actual sleep, mimics what happens in dreamless sleep. Your blood pressure and pulse go down, stress hormones are inhibited, and conscious awareness goes into a more subdued state. Using meditation, you can learn to achieve a "calm in the eye of the storm" sensation by simply taking a five- to twenty-minute break to re-focus and re-balance.

Other Physiological Effects of Meditation

The body relays information through weak electrical impulses from one area to another in conjunction with the environment. The nervous system is the primary conduit, but other parts of the body—the skin, the muscles, and the connective tissues, for example—also conduct electricity. The body's electrical charges flow through negatively and positively charged ions, which relay information with amazing rapidity. Like fans doing the "wave" in a stadium, the ion pathways in the body convey information across the varied systems. It appears that changes produced in the nervous system due to meditation cause changes in other tissues as well. Skin resistance, for example, increases with the practice of meditation and prolonged deep breathing. This suggests that the effects of meditation extend throughout the entire body and are not limited to any particular system.

Most pronounced and beneficial, though, are the effects of meditation on cognitive functioning. Meditation improves concentration and spatial memory, and some studies have shown a correlation between meditation practice and increased performance on standardized testing. Almost everyone has heard about the importance of sleep and a good breakfast before an important exam, but almost no one recommends meditation. While meditation will not replace studying as an aide to exam performance, it can reduce test anxiety and improve concentration. The same benefits would extend to other stressful situations, like going to a job interview or completing a tax return. For people with social anxiety, meditation would be beneficial before going to a party or meeting someone for lunch. Meditation provides a tool for dealing with stressful situations in advance, before they spiral out of control into a panic attack or emotional breakdown. Meditation also improves mental performance, which means that anyone can benefit from it.

Harnessing the Power of Meditation

Meditation provides a great way of reducing the everyday effects of stress, and it can prevent and treat chronic disorders. Here are some of the physiological effects of meditation with deep, slow breathing that have been discussed so far. Meditation:

- Reduces heart rate, blood pressure, and cholesterol
- Lowers oxygen consumption
- Blocks the production of stress hormones
- Fights anxiety and other emotional disorders
- Increases concentration and spatial memory
- Aids in fighting pain

If a pharmaceutical company developed a drug with this many effects, it would quickly make billions of dollars. Meditation is amazing by accomplishing so much for free, using techniques that go back thousands of years. And now, the physiological basis of meditation can be uncovered.

Meditation works by balancing the fight-or-flight response with parasympathetic activity, getting the body to go into a rest and recuperation mode. Meditation induces this resting state through two principle means: slowing the rate of breathing and generating positive thought patterns. With a little bit of instruction and a lot of practice, you can make meditation part of your ongoing regimen for health and well-being.

CHAPTER 3

Meditation Meets Modern Life

Though colonialism brought many ills from Western civilizations to those of the East, the West was subtly transformed by Eastern culture as well. In Europe, translations of literature from China, India, and the Middle East became widely available. As a result, the fundamentals of remote religions and philosophies brought different views of the body, mind, and spirit—views that impressed many Western thinkers.

A Meeting of the Minds

The growth of the global culture in the nineteenth century encouraged the exchange of ideas among diverse traditions. Soon, once-inscrutable traditions of the East became accessible to the West. In 1883, the first World Parliament of Religions was held as part of the Columbian Exposition in Chicago. The event was a landmark in recent religious history: It introduced Eastern philosophy and metaphysics directly to rapt audiences. Hindu, Buddhist, Baha'i, Muslim, Christian, and Jewish speakers joined together to espouse a plan of tolerance and progress among their faiths. As a result, many of those same religious bodies mark that occasion as the migration of their traditions to the world at large, and particularly to English-speaking countries.

QUOTE

"If you win the rat race, you're still a rat."

—Anonymous

One popular, dynamic speaker who made a lasting impression was Swami Vivekananda. A follower of the spiritual teacher Ramakrishna, he introduced the rich heritage of Hinduism to many for the first time. By linking concepts of Western science to ancient teachings, he opened the door to a gradual movement of meditation traditions from the obscure past to modern culture. Others at the parliament demonstrated that, although meditation is found in nearly every religion and culture, it has a distinctive approach in each.

Personality Styles and Meditation

A variety of meditation techniques have developed over time in every society, many adapting to the times and customs of the environment. Other techniques were grafted onto new traditions that have reached us today. One example is the transmission of meditation practices in the Yoga tradition to the Buddhist tradition. In modern times, many of these same techniques have been used in secular settings as well. For instance, many stress-reduction programs offered now incorporate Yoga exercises with Buddhist mental-stillness techniques. In short, meditation techniques from several traditions have joined to become mainstream in meeting the needs of modern living. This is accepted by most of the traditional schools of meditation and encouraged by many teachers. Some techniques may be applicable to certain lifestyles, for instance, although the entire program may not be a perfect fit.

ESSENTIAL

Even though you may not consider yourself a meditator yet, you'll want to choose a meditation program that suits your personality. Exploring the many dimensions of meditation can be satisfying in itself, but taking your attitudes and habits into account can help you discover the best approach.

To start, you will find that there are perhaps as many ways to meditate as there are personality types—no matter what system of classification you use. Let's look at a few of those types, along with their strengths and weaknesses, to help you discover the best way to reach healthy living through meditation.

The Seer

You are intuitive when evaluating something new, first visualizing your involvement before making any decisions. Impressions and dreams are meaningful in the process, and you often pay attention to your hunches. The Seer has strong auditory senses and does well with chant, prayer, and sound support in a meditation practice. Seers make rapid progress in the early stages of meditation but falter once the visual images become stale. In order to receive maximum health benefit from meditation, seers should stretch their capacities by meditating on silence and the ineffable.

The Thinker

You are analytical when presented with new information; an idea has to make sense before you agree to it. You employ a methodical approach when learning a skill and prefer to go by a checklist when performing tasks. The Thinker has a well-developed tactile sense, depending on the sense of touch to balance analytical processes. This ability works well with a meditation practice that employs physical conditioning and sequential development of the body's powers. The self-discipline required for slow, deep breathing, which yields immediate physiological responses in meditation, will come easily to thinkers, but they will have a harder time cultivating feelings of universal good-will necessary to bring meditation to full fruition.

The Executor

You don't like to waste time or energy with nonessentials; getting the job done is what satisfies you the most. Teamwork and feedback are important, and you are not derailed by interferences or delays. The Executor is visually oriented and does well with systems that use images, icons, and symbols. In order to receive maximum stress-reduction from meditation, executors will need to learn to tolerate ambiguity and open-endedness. On the plus side, executors have a strong ability to stay on task, which makes establishing a practice relatively easy.

The Feeler

You enjoy being insulated from the outside world and treasure your own time and space. You will consider new activities if they don't require great adjustments to your lifestyle, and you will seek a few opinions before going ahead. The Feeler has cultivated a gustatory approach to living, appreciating the sensate side of life. A system that includes full-sense involvement, such as ritual meditation, will satisfy this type. The propensity for solitude will make feelers natural meditators, but, for maximum well-being, feelers should coax themselves toward spiritual community to sustain themselves over the long haul.

Tradition or Technique?

In the history of meditation, all approaches can be divided into religious and secular (nonreligious). In short, they fall between the categories of tradition and technique. Now that you have some guidelines on what your type is, you may want to widen your understanding of these approaches and how they can enhance the integration of body, mind, and spirit. This further investigation will also allow you to design your own meditation program, by trial-

and-error and personal preference. First, we will explore the great meditation traditions, because they are the ones we encounter most frequently. Then we will look at the techniques that are found in many of them, and how they can be used independently to achieve the same results as traditional systems.

Tradition

Yoga, Buddhism, Taoism, and other practices are regarded as integrated practices, because they combine religious themes with philosophical approaches, often in the context of the cultural landscapes in which they are practiced. These systems are also viewed as unbroken traditions, because their tenets have been passed without interruption through the ages. However, within these great traditions are also many smaller ones or specialties. These specialties emphasize the use of the mind over the body, for example, or the use of nature and the environment as the vehicles for meditation rather than mental exercises. This concentration doesn't make one specialty superior to another. Rather, it encourages the practitioner to develop different faculties and dimensions.

Technique

The great traditions also convey important precepts of moral development, health and hygiene, and spiritual goals. Stripped of their cultural overtones, these traditions possess great wisdom that can be applied to modern life, and so it is worthwhile to include them in your study. They also make room for the meditator's personal experience as the benchmark for faith and spiritual accomplishment. How else can it be? Since meditation is an inward practice, any results will be derived from your experience rather than an outward, external source.

Once a great deal of Eastern philosophy had filtered into our popular culture, psychologists and physicians recognized certain elements as quite applicable to modern life. They began extracting some of those elements and applying them as techniques for personal improvement with remarkable results. Meditation techniques are almost always found in today's healing, counseling, preventative medicine, and sports and learning programs. They support the goals of each discipline, while offering time-tested benefits for the overall person.

Other derived practices—such as transcendental meditation, insight meditation, and mindfulness meditation—get to the essence of the process without the cultural details. And while some view the origins and details of these practices as important areas of knowledge, it is often necessary to take an expeditious approach. Whether we are dealing with stress, a need for healing, or personal growth, the derived meditation practices are advantageous tools. For those who may have reservations about the cultural or religious peculiarities of a practice, these types of meditation provide intelligent alternatives. And since researchers have examined many of them for their therapeutic value, they are more easily integrated into a personal regimen.

ALERT

Remember that meditation does have a logical progression. Don't try to force yourself to "make it to the next level," or you might find you're not achieving any results. There are no tests, and there is no clear definition of success.

One word of caution is in order here when approaching other cultures. Take the time to get to know the traditions that you encounter: go beyond the surface level familiarity. Study the scriptures and philosophies of the tradition that you want to explore. When visiting retreat and worship centers, make sure to learn the etiquette before arriving. Everyone is a tourist on the spiritual path in some sense, but there are tourists and then there are tourists. When "traveling" through other cultures and traditions, tread lightly. Be curious but not obnoxious, eager but not overeager. Ask questions but phrase them respectfully. And make sure not to take without giving back: even if you don't want to join a particular faith community, you can still help with one of their service projects or other initiatives by volunteering of your time and money.

Science or Art?

You need to know how to approach the process of learning meditation and making it a part of your life. Is meditation a science or an art? Is it logical or creative? Does it fit into your idea of work or play?

If it is a science, then it must have a logical process. There should be a progressive, systematic approach to learning it and applying it in everyday circumstances. And it should also be able to stand up to objective testing through established criteria, such as observing predictable qualities and measuring them.

Meditation does have a logical progression, and you can approach it at your own pace. There are no tests, just your own personal evaluation of the results. The obvious question that arises from this is: What do you want from meditation? Here is a checklist of possibilities:

- **To defuse the stress factors in your life:** You know stress when you experience it, but you don't know how to address it.
- **To regain a sense of well-being:** Even though everything on the outside may appear to be okay, on the inside you don't feel quite right anymore.
- **To understand your inner life:** You recognize your needs and desires, but they remain elusive and difficult to fulfill.
- **To grow to the potential you believe is possible:** You know you are capable of being a better spouse/parent/artist/worker, but things seem to be standing still.

If meditation is an art, then it is a process of self-discovery and expression. It should involve one or more intangible qualities such as emotional and intuitive energies. In this sense, the visual and sensate faculties of our consciousness may stimulate meditation.

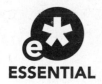

ESSENTIAL

Stress arises from those emotions (such as fear, anger, and frustration) that conflict with your goals. Such emotions always create a division within you, which may be expressed by an inability to complete your responsibilities or achieve your goals. Eventually, the division you feel creates conflict in your relationships and environment.

We should view meditation as both a science and an art. As a science, it features a vast reservoir of techniques that provide viable benefits on many levels: biological, psychological, and spiritual. As an art, meditation provides a do-it-yourself approach to discovering the philosophical and sacred dimensions of our lives. It is the ultimate approach to becoming all we are meant to be.

Your Meditation Goals

Setting realistic goals is an important part of meditation. The following sections highlight some goals that you can work toward. Keep in mind that you'll be striving for them throughout your lifetime; meditation doesn't offer a quick fix. With meditation, you are in charge of your progress, so being realistic is the first step in beginning this practice.

Freedom from Stress

Life is full of stressful conditions, whether you are at work, on vacation, or just doing nothing. Meditation can increase your awareness of when and where stress is to be found, and how to best handle it while being least affected by it. But it can't remove stress completely.

A Positive Attitude

You cannot avoid powerful emotions—positive or negative—unless you are completely removed from the arena of life. Meditation can assist you in discovering your strengths and weaknesses, so you have a solid understanding of yourself. That way, unimportant words and events will have little effect on your true attitude.

Success at What You Do

Whether you are an artist, parent, spouse, or technician, there is always room for improvement. Meditation can help you focus your attention on what you are doing and hone your skills to higher levels. But just as meditation is a continuing process, so is "becoming better."

Enlightenment

Who doesn't want to attain enlightenment? As you go through life, the light becomes brighter when the inner life is developed in unison with the outer life. This is the subtle balance that meditation helps us maintain, but the journey has only begun.

Mind-Body Loops You Can Resolve

One of meditation's primary goals is well-being. But the goal of well-being is common to most people, not just meditators. And we all have our own ideas of what that is, based on our knowledge and experiences. So what prevents us from achieving this goal in our lives? Often, we start chasing attitude "loops" that eventually take over by chasing us. These loops rob us of our sense of well-being. Yes, these are behavior patterns (or psychological syndromes) by another name, but they keep us going back and forth, round and round. Here are some of the mind-body loops that contribute to the loss of well-being.

The Stress-Lethargy Loop

The continual demands of your responsibilities may have you racing to resolve every crisis. This stress is followed by periods of depletion that allow only enough time and energy to recuperate to meet the next demand. In time, it seems that any crisis finds you, and there is no time for relaxing or doing the things you really want to do. Symptoms include overwork and oversleep. If you're often wondering "What if?," you may be caught in the stress-lethargy loop.

The Anxiety-Fear Loop

You may have seen or faced serious disruptions in your life, and they confirmed your worst fears. You expect those disruptions to rear their ugly heads again, and you're not sure you can handle them when it happens. Symptoms include hesitation and restlessness. If you're often worried about the future, you may be stranded in the anxiety-fear loop.

The Panic-Control Loop

You've had everything in your life pretty well managed the way you wanted, but little things seem to be slipping out of your control. The more this happens, the more you try to find ways to get things back in line. Symptoms include feeling overwhelmed and frustrated. If you're asking "Why me?" a lot, you may be in the panic-control loop.

The Anger-Depression Loop

You've had to deal with some menacing people and situations, but you didn't do anything about it. Now you feel defeated and don't know how to break down the brick wall that is blocking your energy. Symptoms include irritability and sluggishness. If you find yourself saying, "No way!" frequently, you may be in the anger-depression loop.

The Bitterness-Isolation Loop

You made it through some difficult times in the past and had to go it alone. You've come to avoid people and places that remind you of that vulnerability, although you'd like it if you could return to the way you used to be. Symptoms include mistrust and lack of motivation. If you find yourself referring to the past frequently, you may be in the bitterness-isolation loop.

FACT

Every day, you absorb a considerable amount of information and impressions from the outside world. Meditation is one way to wring out the sponge, so your experiences don't become stale. It is preventive medicine for the spirit, a refreshing pause for the mind, and a reservoir of calm for the emotions.

Getting out of the Loop with Meditation

So how does meditation address these problematic attitudes? All of these loops have their basis in the sympathetic/parasympathetic balance. Meditation helps you to put a period at the end of the sentence, to hit the "reset" button. The restorative, balancing functions of the parasympathetic system begin to counter-balance the aggressive, active energies of the sympathetic nervous system. On an emotional level, the sense of well-being that derives from internal balance begins to counteract the negative emotions that feed into the loop. Meditation allows you to stop running around the hamster wheel of the loops and regain perspective.

As you examine the different approaches to meditation, you'll notice that certain ideas are emphasized in each system. Here are a few techniques that can help resolve the attitude loops that absorb energy and attention.

Transience. See the inevitable ebb and flow of all things. Problems (and their solutions) are transient: They come and go like the rising and falling tides. When you see this rhythm in life, you're less likely to fall into the stress-lethargy loop.

Compassion. Develop an appreciation of all things. Going through profound life events brings with it a deep feeling for others. When you can express this outlook to others and especially to yourself, anxiety and fear will no longer dominate your feelings.

Surrender. Let go of the mental and emotional attitudes that do not represent you. The more persistently you hang on to them, the more resistant the response from others. By abandoning this approach, you also abandon the panic-control loop.

Detachment. Recognize that you are not attached to conditions that surround you. When you possess objectivity, difficult emotions no longer dictate your actions. This helps you overcome the anger-depression loop.

Unity with Life. Cultivate a rapport with those around you. No matter how different or unfamiliar the territory, discover the qualities you have in common with others. Discovering this unity can remedy the bitterness-isolation loop.

The Language of Meditation

Whether you begin your initial study of meditation on your own or with a teacher, you will encounter certain terms that refer to different qualities and states of meditation. It's not important that you know the meaning of every one, but understanding the general idea will provide you with a guideline. In this way, you will discover through your own experience what the different types and states of meditation mean.

Enlightenment

Enlightenment is the expressed goal of many meditation traditions, such as Yoga and Buddhism. But it may also be the most elusive thing to achieve.

The best way to see this goal is to recognize that we rarely use most of our emotional, intellectual, and physical potential in positive ways. It is as if these areas of our life run on high wattage the way a light bulb does, but the power to illuminate them is very low. When meditation increases the power, these functions "light up," and when all are working in synch, we are "enlightened."

Impermanence

In most meditation traditions, the outer, external reality is viewed as transitory and impermanent. The true reality, the permanent self (superconscious), is uncovered through meditation. When applied to difficult situations, the concept of impermanence helps us see negative experience as inconsequential, not really affecting the permanent dimension of ourselves.

Mindfulness

Mindfulness does not mean mindless or without thought. Rather, it refers to careful observation of the body, emotions, moods, thoughts, and the immediate experience of the meditator. It also includes observation of thought itself. For example, when you look at a picture of a hamburger and milk shake, the idea of hunger may come to mind. Trace that thought to its origin, if possible. Where does it come from? Is it a true sensation from an empty stomach, or a mental picture of a past event, or an emotional picture of feeling satiated?

Nonattachment

Being nonattached does not mean being cut off from others' or one's own senses. Instead, meditation allows us to detach from things that absorb our attention, energy, and vitality long after those efforts are required. By doing this in a constructive way, we can refresh and rejuvenate so our responsibilities become easier to deal with and resolve.

Transformation

Transformation is changing one form of energy into another. We do this constantly, while breathing, eating, and sleeping. Conscious transformation brings attentive thought to the energy you are expending. You then engage your thought, moving it toward the end result of that expenditure, to the results you intend to experience.

CHAPTER 4

Getting Started with Meditation

Meditation is the true wake-up call, providing direct experience in matters of awareness, understanding, and well-being. Reading about meditation can guide you through the labyrinth of self-knowledge, but experience is the only way you can achieve it. Just keep in mind that the meditation experience is meant to be beneficial, but it can become derailed by unrealistic expectations and goals.

Setting the Stage

You can avoid the disappointment that follows the failure to reach unrealistic goals by setting the stage for a meditation practice that you will look forward to. When you're just starting, think of meditation as the creation of your own oasis, a place where you will refresh yourself. When you first think of an oasis, imagine the dry, lifeless terrain surrounding it. That could be the landscape of your work and lack of leisure. You have journeyed for a long time through this region to reach your destination, and now you are approaching it. You may be excited to enter this zone, or perhaps you're relieved. In either case, you've arrived.

Your Meditation Oasis

In the beginning, you will want to select a place where you can begin your meditation practice and continue at your pace, in your own style, without distraction. Ideally this would be a dedicated room or garden for meditation. If you can't dedicate an entire room, try to avoid placing a shrine in a closet or bathroom, because this subconsciously marginalizes your practice. It would be better to partition part of a main room with a screen or furniture. If your meditation space will be located outside, make sure you have a comfortable chair, bench, or cushion, and avoid extremes of heat and cold.

Obviously, a place where interference is at a minimum is ideal. You should find a space where the telephone can be turned off and sounds from other rooms can be shut out.

Electronic and electrical equipment can also be a nuisance. The continual hum of a computer fan or the low buzz of a fluorescent light will be distracting when you are starting to focus your attention inward. Make sure you can easily shut down these machines without jeopardizing your safety or comfort.

Removing Distractions

A cluttered space is a distraction. We are often warned against scattering homework or bills on the dining room table or the bed. This is to avoid contaminating the places where we eat and sleep with reminders of stressful or unpleasant tasks. The same goes for your meditation space. Piles of unopened mail and grocery receipts have their own hypnotic power that you may need to escape. An orderly, clean environment encourages the feeling of readiness and ease.

Most of all, your meditation space should not be a place where foot traffic will disrupt your focus. An area where others will be eating, ironing, or watching television isn't a good choice. Members of your household should not be passing through your space. This will be your sanctuary, so it should offer peace and privacy from the outside world.

Of course, you have to work with the space that you have, and most of us are not lucky enough to have an ideal space to meditate. Complete elimination of distraction is neither possible nor desirable, because the annoying elements in our spaces become grist for the mill of meditation. Behind every distraction is some attachment waiting to be uncovered and diffused, some adjustment in attitude that needs to be made. So strive to have a clean, orderly, inspiring, out-of-the-way place to meditate, but realize that this will never be entirely the case. Even monks and nuns living the cloistered life have physical and mental distractions, which says that these facets of existence can sometimes only be endured or transcended—not eliminated.

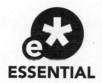

ESSENTIAL

If your space has a window, a natural vista would be helpful for beginning a meditation practice. Trees, bodies of water, and patches of earth are visual aids for "detaching" from thoughts and emotions. Of course, not everyone has the advantage of living near natural sites. You could create one of your own.

Maybe you are fortunate enough to have an exclusive, quiet space that is not frequented by the busy members of your life. Allow as much of the natural environment to prevail. Natural light from one or more windows is valuable. With so many workers performing their tasks indoors in modern times, the sense of nature's rhythms in both the course of the day and the seasons is seriously diminished. This cuts us off from positive influences and the connection with natural life.

Finding the Right Accessories

The meditation environment can reflect your personal tastes and your goals. You can experiment with this, choosing those elements that suit your personality and home décor. No matter what type of meditation you work with—traditional, secular, or your own eclectic version—you'll need some accessories in the beginning and throughout your meditation practice.

Comfort is an important concern. You may be spending some time in this space, and you don't want to be discouraged if it feels uncomfortable. You should be able to maintain a comfortable temperature, and keep a warm blanket or throw nearby in case it gets drafty.

The wall space that surrounds you is another consideration. You may want a blank canvas for your initial meditation practice, or you may feel more at ease with the usual décor. Then again, you may want to choose special wall hangings, a set of favorite prints or a painting. Many meditators pay great attention to such details in their meditation room, but keep in mind that your approach may change. Because you may be experimenting with different meditation styles in the beginning, an elaborate space may change into a simple one in time.

ALERT

Be careful when you choose music. Some sounds can stimulate thinking and memories; others can induce lethargy. You will also want a sound system that allows for continuous play or programmed selections, so you don't have to adjust it continually.

Lighting is another point that you want to resolve. Whether you have access to a lot of natural light or depend on artificial sources, make sure it can be adjusted to minimum and maximum levels. Candles are often used for focus in meditation, but they pose safety problems if not supported securely. Likewise, incense should be burned in containers that will catch the ashes.

Plants and flowers are other additions to the meditation space that can lend a connection to nature and create a fresh atmosphere. You can even use plants as visual reminders of your meditation practice. Each time you water the plants, you will be reminded that you will also need the refreshment of a meditation session. And as the plant grows, so will your proficiency in personal growth and self-awareness.

Music is a big consideration for the beginner. You may want to incorporate background music to get in the mood for meditation, or it may be necessary to balance outside, distracting noises in the dwelling or the street. You can also find useful training tapes and inspirational recordings that are preliminary tools for meditation.

Understanding Body Basics

Successful meditation does not depend on your ability to conform your body to the traditional "lotus" position of the yogi, sitting cross-legged on the floor. But a few guidelines are necessary for productive and comfortable meditation.

Your Spine

First and most importantly, allow your spine to be upright and immobile. This position allows for optimum breathing and less strain on the body overall for maintaining one position over an extended period. Nothing should interfere with circulation. Besides a practice of proper breathing to aid circulation, the right posture ensures that the entire body can oxygenate without hindrance.

For the spine to be upright, you will be either sitting or standing for meditation practice. For now, we will focus on traditional sitting meditation. Which is best: a comfortable chair or the solid surface of the floor?

Sitting postures require a firm foundation, but at the same time, enough padding should be under you to promote circulation and comfort. Few chairs can accommodate the spread of a seated person with folded knees at the sides, so the floor is a good place to begin. However, you may not be able to sit cross-legged for any number of reasons and so a good chair will be necessary.

The second consideration is what to do with your limbs. If you are sitting on the floor, should your legs be crossed or folded? Should your feet be tucked under you or at the side? You'll need to do some experimentation here. And just because someone you know meditates in a perfect, folded leg position doesn't mean you'll be able to do so right away. Keep in mind that circulation is more important than how your position looks.

If you plan to sit in a chair, the same guidelines apply. However, your feet must be supported—either by the floor, a footrest, or a cushion.

Wear comfortable, loose-fitting clothing for meditation, appropriate to the location and occasion. Athletic clothing may be okay in a Yoga class, but it may not be in a temple. When you have found a style or tradition that is likely to "stick," consider investing in garments and tools appropriate to the particular tradition and level of initiation. While clothes and accessories will not buy spiritual insight, they do help to set the tone for the meditation session and should not be disregarded.

Try sitting in several different positions. If, within five minutes, you start to feel numbness in your feet, legs, knees, or bottom, get up and move about for another five minutes. Then try another sitting position. Do this until you find a position that doesn't impose any restrictions or discomfort for at least fifteen minutes at a time.

Your Hands

When you've found your optimum sitting position, what should you do with your hands? You may have seen illustrations of meditating persons with their hands positioned in strange poses; these are called *mudras* (Sanskrit for "signs"). They assist in the meditation by focusing the body as well as the mind. But that is a science for later discovery; for now, you want to decide the most comfortable way to start. If your hands sweat easily, you may want to keep them open, palms up. If they get cold easily, you may want to place them downward, on your lap or knees. Another comfortable position is to place them on your tummy, either folded or interlaced.

Your Eyes

Your eyes are the third consideration: Will they be open or closed? This is another personal preference, and it depends on the environment you've selected as your meditation space. Whether the available light helps you become still and relaxed will determine your choice. However, the eyes-open position is the ideal way to begin meditation, so you don't confuse the practice initially with rest or slumber. Since one of the goals is to raise awareness and harness the mind, using your eyes to notice detail, focus attention, and connect with nature is essential. When groups of people meditate, though, closing your eyes can help avoid the distraction of others around you.

Sitting Postures

The lotus is regarded as the standard sitting posture of meditation. You'll see it depicted in diagrams for the Yoga student, and frequently in Buddhist images from China, Tibet, and Japan. Although it is an accepted way of sitting in the Far East and Middle East, it's not as easily achieved in the West, and that can be a big deterrent when starting a meditation practice. There are variations on this posture though, and everyone can find one that is suitable. Variations on the lotus posture are covered in the following sections, but keep in mind the following caveats before you begin:

- If you choose to sit in a chair, make sure you have a sturdy but comfortable sitting chair with a tall back that will keep your spine straight and your back supported.
- Keep your feet flat on the floor and lean back to rest your neck if necessary.
- Avoid tight clothing or footwear, furniture that pushes against your limbs, and slippery fabric covers that will interfere with comfort and relaxation.
- If you choose to be seated on the floor, make sure the surface is completely flat, using a rug or pad on hard surfaces, followed by a seat cushion or bench that fits you while seated.
- Choose a posture that allows you to place your knees as close to the floor as possible so that your spine will remain upright in a beneficial position.
- If your back tires easily, you can lean against a wall with your legs stretched out in front of you.

For sitting meditation, the lotus posture is viewed as the ideal way to connect the body with the vital energy of earth. Like a lotus, your trunk is akin to the flower's root, grounding itself to the stabilizing force of the land. At the same time, the watery regions of thought and emotion surround you, yet the meditation process enables you to float through them unaffected.

Burmese Lotus

The Burmese lotus is so named because it is the sitting tradition of Southeast Asia. The legs are folded, one in front of the other, so that the calves and feet of both legs are resting on the floor. This is a good beginning posture.

Half and Quarter Lotus

For the half lotus, while seated, just one leg (whichever is more comfortable) is folded upward to rest on the opposite inner thigh. The other leg is tucked under the first. This position takes some practice.

ESSENTIAL

The keys to comfortable standing meditation are standing upright and maintaining balance. If you become tired, lean your back fully against a wall. Then you can conclude the meditation session.

The quarter lotus is similar to the half lotus, except that instead of resting on the thigh, one leg is resting on the calf of the opposite leg. This posture is easy to negotiate.

Full Lotus

While seated, the legs are folded upward, with the right foot placed on the left hip and the left foot placed on the right hip. The hands rest on the knees. An advanced version of this posture is the *Baddha Padmasana*, where the hands are crossed behind the back and the big toes on either side are grasped. Your chin is then pressed down and your eyes are focused on the tip of the nose. This posture is not recommended for beginners.

Standing Meditation

You may find yourself at a time or place where traditional sitting meditation is not possible. If that should be the case, standing meditation is quite effective, although it may not be comfortable for extended periods. Any meditation lasting less than fifteen minutes is adaptable to standing meditation.

FACT

> When sharing space with a roommate or family members, you may want to arrange your meditation time when you will not likely be interrupted. When one individual in a group starts a meditation practice, it often influences others to follow suit, at least in spirit. Quiet time is valuable to all, and it is beneficial to share in the flow of reflection and peace that meditation brings.

Stand with your spine upright and your shoulders straight. This isn't a military stance, because that would be tiring. Instead, your shoulders should be evenly balanced on both sides. Your chin is tilted slightly upward but not stretched. Stand with your feet about twelve inches apart, far enough to balance your weight evenly. Your hands may be placed with palms against your thighs. Or you may find it more comfortable to hold both hands close to the center of your body, palms inward. Do not cross or fold your arms.

Prone Meditation

Prone meditation is also called lying meditation and in Yoga, *shavasana*, or the Corpse. Despite the eerie name, this posture makes it possible to maintain mental and physical stillness while lying down.

Start by choosing a firm surface. If you're on the floor, make sure it is padded enough not to press against portions of the body and cause numbness. If the surface is too comfortable, such as a mattress, it may encourage lethargy and sleep. Try to find a happy medium.

Lie flat on your back, with your spine touching as much of the floor surface as possible. Relax your neck and shoulders, and allow your arms to relax with open palms about six inches away from your body. Look directly up without stretching your neck in any way. If the light from the ceiling is too strong, use a floor lamp instead.

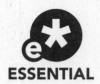

ESSENTIAL

Make arrangements to deal with unexpected interruptions. Set your phone on silent. Make sure the cat is out, the dog is in—or the birdcage is covered.

Finding the Right Time to Meditate

When is a good time for meditation? The diurnal (daily) clock is the one we set our conscious life to, but few are aware of the subtle forces at work each day. At sunrise, the environment is illuminated and natural life awakens. Depending on the time of year and geographic location, the sun may begin to warm earth, and the temperature arouses certain animal species to either come out into the light or retreat. At noon, the sun is directly overhead, and with light and heat at their most intense. Midday is a vital time, and the life force is at its peak. At sunset, the light diminishes as it sinks below the horizon and most active life begins to withdraw. The midnight hour is also a pivotal time of the day, although few are awake to appreciate it.

These four periods are regarded as the "peak points" of the day, the diurnal rhythm. The sun is either on one of the horizons (east or west), the midheaven (at noon), or the nadir (at midnight). This is how it is viewed both astronomically and in astrology, although each has a different perspective on the meaning. But both agree that these peak points are the vital times of the day and influence human behavior in profound ways.

So when should you meditate? Actually, the peak points of the day are when you are most ambitious and may want to practice, but these times often conflict with other duties.

Many people find it most useful to start the day with a morning meditation. By clearing the mind and consciously experiencing stillness, the day does not seem so daunting or ordinary—whichever the case may be. An early evening meditation similarly stills and clears the mind of the day's events.

Whatever time you find best fits your schedule; try to keep it away from mealtimes. If you have not eaten for several hours, a growling stomach may interrupt your meditation session. And if you're meditating right after a meal, the digestive process could similarly be disruptive. Besides, sitting for an extended period right after eating tends to compress the esophagus, bringing on acid reflux or heartburn.

FACT

Some Yoga texts say that the two hours before sunrise are optimum for deep meditation. Not everyone is able or willing to make the switch to early morning hours, but try it at least once. A vacation time, pilgrimage, or retreat may make it possible. It also helps to form the intention to arise at a specific time just before falling asleep the night before.

Knowing How Long to Meditate

There are conflicting guidelines on the length of a session depending on the meditation system in question, so in the beginning it's up to you to decide. Some recommend forty-five minutes; others say that twenty minutes is enough of a meditation break to make a difference.

Setting a timer or placing a clock in your meditation space may be useful in the beginning, but you don't want the clock to rule your session. In fact, the passage of time is always monitored by the subconscious mind. In meditation, this awareness often comes forward. So, set yourself up mentally for a fifteen-minute meditation session, and stop when you think you've achieved it. If not, try it again the next time you have a session. Since meditation is a process of becoming aware, the passage of time will make itself known soon enough. Remember, you are leaving the world of schedules and moving into the timeless.

Once you have decided on meditation timing, you must commit to following it consistently. There may be times when this is not possible, though after a while you will find yourself able to meditate at any time and, eventually, any place. Remember that this is only a commitment to yourself, and not to any one person or long-term goal. It's a gift of time that you are investing in your well-being.

Practicing One-Breath Meditation

Everyday life continually poses challenges to our inner peace. In the midst of a stressful episode, whether at home or at work, we often long for the peaceful moments that a secluded, quiet meditation offers. But the real world doesn't offer such moments when they're most needed. We have to create them. At these times, a conscious pause can refresh the body and mind just as well as an extended meditation session. All that's needed is the desire to stop and take action—or no action as the case may be.

ALERT

If you're squeezing meditation in between daily responsibilities, you aren't allowing enough time for a good practice. Waking up an extra fifteen minutes early could remedy that, or moving errands to just one part of the day instead of scattering them throughout the day could ease up on the time crunch.

If you find yourself at a standstill at work, feeling that you've come to the end of the rope you're climbing, stop. Remind yourself that this is an opportune time for momentary meditation, to refresh and relax your mind from the climb. Pause all thoughts and remind yourself that your inner peace prevails at this moment. Think of that peace as a place within you. Straighten your spine as you do this, and lift your chin upward. Focus your eyes above your head, at the ceiling or wall. Take a conscious breath, slowly and deliberately. Think of your place of peace opening its door as the air fills your lungs. On exhaling, appreciate the moment for allowing you to pause, and return to the work at hand.

CHAPTER 5

Experiencing Meditation

Meditation begins with a very simple premise—focusing your attention on a single point. Meditation trains the overactive mind to slow its frenetic pace and hold awareness still. The focus of meditation could be the breath, a chakra, or an image of a deity, but, no matter what the focal point, the goal is to quiet the mind.

Thoughts and Feelings

Once you begin to focus your attention, a host of interesting situations—in the realm of thoughts and feelings—present themselves. Thoughts and feelings are important considerations in the early stages of meditation. As soon as you establish your time and space and start your first sessions, you may become aware that thoughts and feelings begin to rush forward for your attention. Everything you may have put on the back burner comes forward, seeking attention or resolution.

Handling Thoughts

Instead of trying to push thoughts out of the way, you could make a meditation of viewing them in a detached, disengaged manner. You can do this by neutralizing them. Here's how it works: If a distracting thought comes forward, welcome it and ask it to put its case before you. Then listen to what it communicates and return it to the back burner. Do not personify the thought; view it as a disembodied object, like a bubble or cloud. Consider what the thought communicated to you for only a moment, giving it a minimal amount of time, and allow the next thought to come forward.

QUOTE

"To God, everything is beautiful, good, and just; humans, however, think some things are unjust and others just."

—Heraclitus

For example, you are initiating a new meditation and the thought comes to your mind that you didn't shop for dinner. Ordinarily, you might think of a quick menu, the items you'll need, and if they're not in the kitchen, where to buy them. That might lead to remembering that your checkbook is at the office, so you'll have to use the credit card, and the bill arrived yesterday.

Instead, you neutralize the thought by acknowledging that dinner wasn't included in today's planning. Tell the thought: I will plan it when my meditation is over. Give the thought your attention, assign it a place, and move on.

Focusing Emotion

Feelings are a different matter, arising from another realm of our being. Emotions are not amenable to logic; they possess a stream of action all their own. We can visualize thought as linear and emotion as circular. Thus, we cannot reason with or analyze feelings. The impressions we receive from feelings, however, do not have to affect our awareness.

Feelings may come through the body as sensations, pleasant or unpleasant. They may also appear as attitudes, especially toward yourself. For example, as you begin to sit in meditation, you feel restless, saying to yourself, "Okay, let's get down to business." What does this mean?

Initially, you may feel a wave of impatience, because you procrastinated throughout the day and it's weighing on you. Then you may feel a wave of frustration, reminded that there doesn't seem to be enough time to do everything you want. And finally, a sense of anger may well up, because the interference of others has taken up so much of your time.

Instead, address the impatience with humor. "What's the hurry? I'm here to be free of business." Likewise, meet the frustration with calm. "The time I give myself will multiply the time I can give to everything else." And always neutralize anger with kindness. "I have been inconvenienced by the interference of others, but now I can make it up to myself." Other feelings may appear when you begin to meditate (for example, hopelessness, discouragement, and other counterproductive feelings). What would you say to a close friend who expressed those feelings to you? You would undoubtedly extend words of hope, encouragement, and motivation. You are no different than your friends.

Countering emotions is not the aim here, as that can be conflicting. The goal is to balance and settle the emotions—and this is not a quick, easy task. You will need much practice at this, because you are probably harder on yourself than anyone else. One attitude to always keep throughout this process is what the Dalai Lama, Tibet's spiritual leader, calls "loving kindness." You must practice it on yourself in the beginning, and it should be the byword during all the time you spend in meditation.

Alternating Thought and Feeling

Thought and feeling can take their turns in sessions. Devote one session to thought, the next to feeling. You may alternate each time you sit for a meditation. As you continue this pattern, an interesting phenomenon begins to happen. The rush of thoughts and feelings subside, and you begin to notice that something else is present—your own awareness, anticipating the next thought or feeling. At that moment, there is a pause in thought and feeling, and it is that pause that you are seeking to cultivate. That is meditation.

Asking questions is a beneficial exercise in noticing thoughts and feelings through meditation. This is not a process of analyzing. Rather, it is a way of exercising mindfulness, one of the qualities sought in meditation. And throughout the process, you are also bringing forth another innate ability: insight. Together, these dormant tools can provide you with honest, clear answers to all the questions you may have about yourself and your life in general.

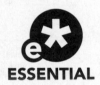

ESSENTIAL

All forms of meditation have many teachings and goals in common: to be in the moment, to establish a distance between your self and your thoughts and feelings, and to become, metaphorically, the anchor. The rest of you is the ship, and your surroundings are the sea.

While you are in meditation, thoughts and feelings present themselves. Don't let them fly away; catch them—like butterflies—and ask the following questions:

- Why do I think/feel this way about that person or situation?
- What causes led to this thought/feeling?
- Why do I still think/feel this way about that person or situation?
- What conditions could make this thought/feeling change?

This is an exercise in "mental housecleaning." And like regular housecleaning, you can observe yourself doing it. Layers of awareness unfold like the proverbial lotus, and you experience insights along the way.

Seed Meditation

It's easy to see how there can be many types of meditation for different goals and different people. Every culture and religion has a meditative tradition, and some approaches continue to evolve today, as offshoots of older, established traditions.

Even so, there are still some approaches that apply to everyone's choice of meditation style. Starting with a view of those will steer you toward the goal of establishing a meditation practice that suits you. Essentially there are two ways that meditation can be practiced: "with seed," and "without seed." These are generic terms, and just about every type of meditation will fall into one of these two approaches.

Meditation with Seed

What is meditation with seed? Here, a single image, word, or sound is employed to focus the mind in order to reach the launching point away from ordinary mental activity. In some religious traditions, certain prayers serve as seed meditations. They can be quite extensive, and the entire meditation practice may be based on recitation or the silent reading of such prayers or revered writings. In others, words of power or mantras are repeated at length to attain the launching point. These may be short or long; they may be repeated several times or just once, to arouse or stimulate the mind to reach the launching point.

Seed meditation can also direct the meditator's focus to images or sounds. The visual and auditory concentration helps the practitioner stay within a theme or atmosphere of meditation. Some traditions emphasize this through meditation or prayer with statues, illustrations, and architectural design. Others use music, sounds with bells or drums, chants, and spoken prayers.

Meditation Without Seed

Meditation without seed is another technique that is valued in some traditions. Here, the goal is to empty the mind of all its conscious and unconscious contents. The senses are also muted with stillness. This can be accomplished through silence, separation from familiar surroundings, and elimination of all but the basic necessities of daily existence. Monastic life and retreats are an example of this type of meditation tradition. Through this, a very powerful launching point may be attained, far above the ordinary realm of conscious thought or appearances. Naturally, meditation without seed is an advanced form, and the beginner is encouraged to begin exercises with seed to strengthen mental focus.

The Value in Both Techniques

Either approach—with or without seed—is quite effective, depending on the circumstances and the practitioner. The advantage of seed meditation is that it allows the familiar to become so familiar that we no longer even think about it. In fact, we are released from thinking altogether. The advantage of meditation without seed is that it dispenses with the tendency to focus on familiar things, so other realities can be discovered.

The use of seed meditation is expressed in a number of modern paths, although it is called by other names. It may be referred to as intentional meditation, where specific goals are formulated and the meditation experience is aimed toward those ends. This path includes guided meditations, in which the goals may be quite temporary, but the meditator is "guided" by a teacher or meditation leader. Meditation without seed is also referred to as choiceless meditation, a term coined by Jeddu Krishnamurti, a twentieth-century philosopher and proponent of self-discovery through meditation.

ALERT

Giving yourself time for rest between exercises is very important in meditation. Reflecting on your immediate actions and reactions are meditative exercises in themselves.

The analogy of a seed, however, is most appropriate. It alludes to the "unfolding" of the conscious mind to reach enlightenment, just as a seed grows to a flower and unfolds its splendid petals to reveal a perfect design. At the same time, a seed resides within the mature plant, indicating that another flower, or level, awaits unfolding in the future.

The Right Way to Breathe

Have you ever listened to your breathing? Or observed your rhythm of inhaling and exhaling? Most people who do so find that they breathe in short breaths that do not completely fill the lungs. Once they notice, they start to take deeper breaths. The infusion of oxygen by this exercise can bring on a "high" of sorts, but after a while they forget the deep breathing and go off to their regular activities with unmonitored, shallow breathing.

ESSENTIAL

When practicing breathing, you may get a "goose bump" sensation on your forearms or running down your spine. This response, called piloerection, comes from the changing electrical impulses in the body as a result of deep breathing. Don't be alarmed if this does or does not happen: it is just something to notice along the way.

Of course, we take air into the body through the nose and mouth. But meditation masters say that the "center" where we are drawing in the air should not be in our nostrils, or throats, or even the lungs. Rather, we should breathe in from the stomach, the way babies breathe.

Breathing Warm-Ups

If you are ready to pursue the goal of a personal meditation practice, then getting started with some exercises can set the foundation for your regimen right away. Let's start—as most meditation training starts—with breathing.

You may wonder why breathing is a central component in meditation and why it is emphasized so much. After all, breath is a natural, autonomic function of the body. But that's why it's so important. When the body is completely at rest, breathing becomes quite noticeable—at times, it even intrudes into awareness of the present. Centuries ago, the rhythm, strength, and energetic exchange of breath with the body was recognized as the ideal timekeeper and modulator. There's no escaping it, and there's every reason to use breathing consciously and optimally, because it contributes so much to physical and mental relaxation. Needless to say, you should use good breathing habits, which you can promote with a few warm-up exercises.

Standing Breath

Stand with your feet slightly apart to balance your weight. Focus only on your breathing for three minutes. Do not attempt to control or direct your breath; just observe it.

Now take three "good" breaths, not necessarily deep or long but comfortably filling your lungs as you inhale and exhale. As you take in each breath, raise your arms; then lower them as you exhale. While inhaling, think of the air also entering your body from the ground upward to your head. Try to allow each breath equal time in duration and quality. And try to keep the rhythm the same as your "normal" breathing, especially in the beginning.

Sitting Breath

Sit in a comfortable chair, making sure that you are as upright as possible and your feet are comfortably on the floor. Place your hands on your lap or palms down on your thighs. Focus only on your breathing for three minutes. Do not attempt to control or direct your breath; just observe it.

Next, lower your head to your chest, and inhale while slowly raising your head. As you exhale, lower your head back to your chest. Do this for three "good" breaths. Try to do it as slowly as possible.

ALERT

Go slowly. Don't set any specific goals or expectations. It's still too early for that. If you can't do the exercise in the time or manner you planned, look forward to the next opportunity to continue your development.

Body Warm-Ups

Physical sensation is one of the first things you will become aware of in meditation. When they are not in motion, your senses are directed inward, rather than outward, and you will notice things that may not have been apparent at other times. Therefore, you need to relax physically as much as possible before a meditation session, so you aren't distracted by body stress.

Spinal Stretch

To help the spine maintain a natural, upright position, start with a good stretch. Lie down on the floor on your stomach, face turned to the side. Take three relaxed breaths. Then, with your hands on either side of you pushing against the floor, lift the top half of your body off the floor, arching your back in the process. Stretch upward slowly, turning your head forward and stretching your chin toward the ceiling. Don't force your back into a strenuous stretch or lift your torso for an extended period. Just try it to see how comfortably your back can arch into a good stretch. Lower yourself back to the floor and take another three relaxed breaths.

FACT

Meditation, like medicine, is a practice. It requires time and patience and, most of all, dedication. Practice makes perfect—and in this case, the perfection you seek already resides within. Meditation is the key to discovering that wonderful resource.

Leg Stretch

Sitting for an extended period can be difficult if you are not acclimated to it. As you work on sitting for longer periods of time, stretch your legs at pre-determined intervals to encourage proper circulation. This stretching may be used as a warm-up and as a "break" in meditation, especially in the beginning. It also helps strengthen the lower vertebrae in the back.

Lie down on the floor on your back, arms at your side and hands palm downward. Take three relaxed breaths. On the third breath, lift one leg; bend it, bringing the knee toward your chest. Use both hands to grasp your bent leg and bring it as close to your chest as comfort allows. Take three relaxed breaths, and on the third breath release your bent leg and allow it to return to the floor. After allowing a minute for circulation, repeat the stretch with the other leg.

Working with a Teacher

Gurus, lamas, swamis, and spiritual guides—it's not hero worship, but it's easy to see how that feeling can develop while looking for a meditation teacher. The complicated history of spirituality as it spread from its various sources has contributed to this uncertain relationship between preceptor and student.

Spirituality had been a perplexing matter of dogma, faith, and social acceptance in the West for centuries, often controlled by the ruling elite or government. With the founding of democratic states came freedom of religion, and for most it was a tentative foray out of the closet of orthodoxy. Unfortunately, the situation did not just apply to religious belief and practice. Practically the entire realm of spirit—including philosophy, psychology, and metaphysics—was relegated to the back burner of popular culture. When accomplished practitioners of various meditation traditions came to the West throughout the twentieth century, the public was either beguiled or confused by their mystery and charisma.

Understand the Culture

Certain cultural beliefs are woven into the great meditation traditions. A novice meditator must understand these beliefs before making a commitment to enter a training program as a student or disciple with a teacher or master. In Eastern countries, centuries of tradition are incorporated in the custom of discipleship. The teacher accepts the student and imparts the sum of his or her knowledge to that pupil. This process often takes many years and requires a complete commitment in time and loyalty.

In many cases, more than study is required. The novice may tend to the teacher's needs by running errands, cooking, and cleaning the learning environment. These duties are considered a privilege for the student and a profound responsibility for the teacher. In this system, much is taught that does not involve book learning or memorizing. The student learns practical lessons through everyday experience, such as tending a garden or brewing a pot of tea.

The advantage is that the student earns the right to the teacher's exclusive knowledge and talents, and that extends into the future when the student becomes a teacher in his own right. And for the teacher, passing on personal and accumulated talents is the fulfillment of a life's work. However, a pupil is limited by the knowledge and experience of the teacher. So if you choose to study meditation with one teacher, you must have some idea of what you want and what the teacher can offer.

ALERT

With the widespread availability of meditation training, it's not necessary to make a lifetime commitment to a particular teacher or tradition to gain the benefits of that practice. Few masters will present themselves that way; if they do, you should question the veracity of the program.

Know the Costs

Should a reliable, comprehensive meditation program require a substantial investment in either time or money? This is a question every beginner wants answered, yet, amazingly, is reluctant to ask. Realistically, specialized training in any self-improvement program is going to require a financial investment. Here are some reasonable expenses that should be covered by students:

- Rent for a reserved space in a room, school, or center
- Overhead costs such as janitorial service and utilities
- The teacher's time (salary)
- Costs of printed materials, books, and audiotapes or videotapes
- Transportation costs for the teacher

If you are asked to donate an unspecified amount to cover your meditation program, take these expenses into account and pay accordingly. Some teachers are very dedicated and live solely on the income they obtain from their students.

Question any requests for specified amounts of money that will be applied to unspecified expenses. For example, a $100 request for the "building fund" should be voluntary and tax-deductible.

Seeking out Meditation Communities

In the tradition of the great meditation schools of the Near and Far East, some communities—spiritual, contemplative, devotional—offer meditation training. Some offer short retreats, a few days away from the outside world, which are useful for the busy person. Other schools offer extended training periods, perhaps for a month or more, to develop specific meditation techniques. Students who attend these courses may receive certification or initiation in the discipline. Although you may not intend to teach meditation technique in the near future, training events are a way to acquire a comprehensive view. As you put the information into practice, you will appreciate the depth of experience that you acquired at longer sessions.

Retreats are another opportunity to experience meditation under the guidance of one or more leaders. A single retreat can advance your practice better than several months of practice in everyday life. Organized retreats surround you with all the components of meditation, even if you have been unable to establish them in your regular life. Quiet time, peaceful surroundings, well-selected music and readings, and people of like mind create the experience. Everyone should experience a retreat at least once.

Ashrams and monasteries often open their facilities to part-time residents. Preparing the community's food, caring for the living quarters, and completing tasks in the library or school are activities that are expected of the student in addition to worshipping, studying, and meditating. The retreat attendant becomes part of the discipline of the community and leaves a different person than the one who entered. If you are looking for a place to take a retreat, do an Internet search for "monastery," "ashram," or "retreat" along with the name of the desired state or region. You should be able to find a facility nearby. If this doesn't work, consider going on a solitary retreat in a park or national forest.

Teaching Others

Whether you have studied some of the great traditions, have had some experience with life in a meditation community, or have done neither, you are never truly a "beginner." Everyone has some experience in meditation, either through deliberate effort or circumstance.

But if you become seriously interested in teaching meditation to others, progressive training or mentorship is the best way to prepare for the work. Such training should include assisting the teacher with other students, developing your own style, and mastering as many techniques of the "school" as possible.

ALERT

Don't allow yourself to be coerced into signing up for progressive meditation training. Remember, this is a realm in which experience is the key to advancement, not the number of books read or tapes purchased.

You should also be familiar with some terminology you'll hear along the way, including the following terms, all of which are Sanskrit, though many are used interchangeably in Yoga and in Buddhist organizations:

- **Ashram ("effort"):** In Hinduism, a group that follows a particular spiritual discipline. A guru or teacher guides the disciples or students. The ashram is usually removed from everyday life and is modeled after an ascetic, simple existence.
- **Sangha ("crowd"):** In Buddhism, the group of practitioners who follow a teacher. In particular, Sangha refers to the body of teachers and followers who form the Buddhist community (one of the three jewels). The Sangha is not attached to any specific place.
- **Satsang ("good company"):** This term refers to a gathering of mutually supportive students or seekers of wisdom, a Yoga community that is not attached to a particular ashram.

Learning meditation with groups or communities can be a rewarding experience, but consider the following points when you are making the choice:

- Know exactly what the course of study or activity will entail. A program outline should be available, and it should clearly explain what will be presented and when.
- Be fully informed of the costs and responsibilities. All fees should be listed, and extras should be explained (such as "private room").

- If certain duties are required, you should be informed before you arrive. You do not want to be surprised with new or unfamiliar duties while you are there.
- Understand your living arrangements. If you are to share space with roommates, you must know that selection will be made based on your criteria and not someone else's. Likewise, sharing a bathroom or kitchen with a group of people may have other considerations, so be prepared.
- Be clear about rules and regulations. Talking, exercising, and chewing gum may be okay or strictly forbidden. Don't be shy about asking, either; you may be called on later to advise someone who is more in the dark than you are.
- Always ask what is customary for clothing and diet. You do not want to be self-conscious when everyone is wearing a kimono and you are in sweatpants.

In the final analysis, it's not necessary to look for an expert to guide you when you are starting a meditation practice. There are a number of basic steps you can take on your own to start and develop the habit of meditation. Ultimately, the process begins and ends with you.

CHAPTER 6

A Meditation Science

We all want to remove ourselves from the mental pressures that incessantly beg for attention. So when we do have moments of freedom from thought, we may be surprised at what we encounter—a growling stomach, a sore foot, a pain in the neck. Why didn't we notice these things before?

The Yoga Tradition

Meditation has a few surprises in store for you. To begin with, the stillness of the mind sharpens your senses, so you will become aware of things that your everyday consciousness tends to minimize. The most important of these is the body, and this has a considerable impact in the world of meditation. The body becomes the instrument par excellence for communicating with your inner self. But first, it has to be "finely tuned," or at least trained in the basics of relaxation and calm.

There is more to Yoga than stretching your body into contorted positions in order to attain peace of mind. Yoga is an integrated system, a philosophy of life with a rich body of wisdom. It provides guidelines for thinking, action, diet, healing, and relationships. In short, Yoga is a comprehensive approach to living that may take a lifetime to master. But the rewards affect every dimension of life, not just the spiritual. The root meaning of Yoga suggests "yoking" or "uniting." In essence, it is the art of becoming integrated with the source of life.

Although it predates Hinduism, Yoga is strongly rooted in the ancient religion of India that still dominates the region with 470 million followers. There are an additional 300,000 practitioners of Hinduism in North America. Its essential doctrine is the cyclic rebirth of the soul, in human or animal form. The cycle is believed to continue until the soul attains enlightenment with the source of its creation. There is no formal clergy, but gurus ("teachers") of various approaches and techniques are acknowledged with respect and community support.

Yoga has a rich source of teachings that are among the oldest in the world. The most ancient Hindu texts are collectively known as the Vedas, a very large body of writings written in Sanskrit from 1500 to 1200 B.C.E. The Vedas are divided into four sections: the Rig-Veda (poetry), the Sama-Veda (philosophy), the Yajur-Veda (sacrificial texts), and the Atharva-Veda (mystical ceremony). The knowledge contained in the Vedas is believed to have been revealed to the rishis ("ancient seers") through deep meditation.

The foundation for Yoga and its diverse techniques arose from the Vedic literature. Meditation is an essential component of Hinduism's goal: the quest for enlightenment and union with the source of creation. But it is viewed as just one ingredient in a multifaceted formula for attaining a full life.

The primary Hindu deities are not celestial images of worship. Though often seen in Hindu temples and sculpture, the deities represent universal principles embodied in the natural forces that compose all material life. They are also used as images of meditation, becoming the foci for contemplation and wisdom. The most important is the Trimurti ("form of three"), the Hindu trinity. In some religious iconography, the Trimurti is pictured as a single body with three heads, each looking in a different direction.

The chief deity of the Trimurti is Brahma, the creator. He embodies the passions and desires that brought the phenomenal world into being. He is the source, the beginning, and the path of return.

The second deity is Vishnu, the preserver, who represents the principle of maintenance. He embodies the powers of mercy and compassion, which maintain the world. In Hindu belief, Vishnu reincarnates as Krishna and Rama, great folk heroes who guided others and attained divine status.

FACT

Yoga ("to yoke") has become a buzzword in modern Western society. It is viewed as a practice that promotes peace of mind, a flexible body, and a host of other positive benefits sought as a remedy to our stressful lifestyles. Yoga has also become the most widespread exercise program in the West since its introduction at the turn of the twentieth century.

The third figure is Shiva, the destroyer, who embodies the principle of rage and destruction. Though some may see Shiva as adverse and negative, Hinduism views this principle as a necessary component in the life of the universe.

While cult worship of the deities continues in India to this day, Hindu scholars view these figures as metaphors for the phenomenal world. In other words, Hindu cosmology sees the universe as consisting of these three forces: creation, preservation, and destruction. Every material form in existence is composed of these forces and subject to them as well. In Yoga practice, this is a fundamental concept from which meditation, healing, diet, and hygiene arise.

Other important deities include Kali, the Shakti ("consort" or feminine half) of Shiva. She is the dark force of primeval energy and sorcery. Though destructive, Kali also "clears the path" for the aspirant, periodically bringing order to chaos. Ganesha is the elephant-headed deity who grants wisdom and removes obstacles from the path of the seeker. He is patron of scholars and astrologers in India. Lakshimi, the consort of Krishna, is a benevolent deity governing motherhood, fortune, and happiness.

The Eight Limbs of Yoga

On the philosophic side, the Vedic sage Patanjali (ca. 200 B.C.E.) penned the oldest discourses on Yoga. In them, he presented methods for attaining enlightenment, emphasizing the use of mind and body in very practical ways. His teaching, the *Yoga Sutra,* outlines eight branches or "limbs" of Yoga practice that represent stages of physical, moral, and spiritual progression. These branches help define the goals of Yoga and provide guidelines for practice and improvement. The first four branches address physical and emotional life; the next four emphasize the use of mental powers.

FACT

A guru ("teacher") is a spiritual master in either the Yogic or Buddhist traditions. There are four levels of the guru: the student's parents, the teacher of a trade or means of livelihood, the spiritual teacher, and the cosmic master who is discovered through enlightenment. A swami ("respected sir") is an accomplished master of a particular Yoga teaching.

The eight limbs of Yoga are really guideposts along the path of human progress. If you look at the plan, it clearly outlines a process for refining mind and body in order to approach the realm of spirit. Beginning with the *yamas* and *niyamas,* the directives point to the development of morals and values (the emotional level). The *asanas* and *pranayamas* then provide discipline and vitality to the body (the physical level). Next, *pratyahara* and *dharana* develop the mind to its fullest potential (the mental level). And at the pinnacle of this system, *dhyana* and *samadhi* bring the practitioner into harmony with her innate powers and those of the universe (the level of spirit). These rules and their characteristics are:

- **Yamas ("restraints" or "abstentions"):** Injunctions that are intended to eliminate negative human qualities. These are presented as goals of practice in thought, word, and deed. There are five *yamas*.
- **Niyamas ("observances" or "purifications"):** Ethical guidelines intended to guide the practitioner toward a moral life. There are five *niyamas*.
- **Asanas ("postures"):** The form of Yoga most people are familiar with. The physical postures are meant to align the body with its natural powers and assist in concentration and control. The physical as well as the spiritual benefits are important, because both represent the outcome of enlightenment. There are many forms and sets of *asanas*.
- **Pranayama ("breath"):** The science of breath control. Here, the simplest, most natural function becomes a vehicle for physical and mental transformation. There are many techniques for practicing *pranayama* under different circumstances.
- **Pratyahara ("withdrawal"):** The practice of drawing the consciousness inward. The process emphasizes differing techniques for separating conscious thought from the external senses in order to prepare the mind for greater uses.
- **Dharana ("concentration"):** The science of focusing the mind into a kind of "one-pointedness." Here, it is possible, among other things, to naturally awaken the body's inherent life force. This branch also teaches visualization and affirmation to accentuate healing and purification processes in the body.
- **Dhyana ("meditation"):** Once concentration is achieved, the mind attains a stillness. Its goal is to reach the stage of awareness, in which the practitioner is fully aware of his body's presence (feelings, instincts) without restraints or control.
- **Samadhi ("absorption"):** The ultimate goal of Yoga, divine rapture. As the meaning implies, the individual identity is absorbed into identity with the infinite source of life. This level is viewed as the fullest possible state of consciousness.

The Five Yamas

The *yamas* are the first stage of Yoga practice and set the course for individual progress. Remember that they are attitudes for cultivation; the process of striving is as valuable as the actual achieving in this stage. The *yamas* include:

- **Ahimsa ("nonviolence"):** To avoid inflicting injury even at the expense of personal exposure to injurious situations. This was the basis of Mahatma Gandhi's philosophy of nonviolence.
- **Aparigraha ("nonattachment"):** To separate oneself from all possessions, material and mental. This is a very tall order, one that you can only strive for. Attachments stem from cravings, and at most we can only distance ourselves from those that serve only to perpetuate themselves.
- **Asteya ("nonstealing"):** To avoid thievery, covetousness, and jealousy. These attitudes promote inflammatory feelings, such as aggravation and bitterness.
- **Brahmacharya ("moderation"):** To control the external senses through moderate living. This injunction is understood in several ways—purity in association with others, the practice of chastity for the unmarried, and celibacy for those dedicated to spiritual enlightenment.
- **Satyam ("truthfulness"):** To express goodness through truthful interaction with others. However, telling the truth involves more than social honesty. Making the effort to remove self-deception and erroneous assumptions contributes to truthful living.

ESSENTIAL

Yoga is the path or means to unify the passions or physical self with the *buddhi*, or higher mind. There are a variety of approaches to accomplishing this, each representing one of the paths or "schools" of Yoga.

The Five Niyamas

The *niyamas* ("observances") are the second stage of Yoga practice. They are qualities that compliment the *yamas* and represent the goals of virtue for the practitioner. The *niyamas* include:

- **Shaucha ("purity"):** The techniques for internal and external cleanliness for both body and mind. The body is not viewed as unclean in Yoga practice. Rather, it is seen as being continually exposed to conditions that taint its innate beauty. The effort to be aware of those conditions is part of this observance.

- **Santosha ("contentment"):** Refers to satisfaction with the realities that the practitioner faces and accepts. Acceptance is very important in meditation because it eliminates feelings of frustration and regret. Self-acceptance is even more important because it allows for awareness and growth.

- **Tapas ("austerity"):** Includes struggle and stringent behavior but also the practice of intense spiritual exercises that prepare the practitioner for ethical progress. What does this mean? Self-discipline and doing without some of the "extras" are always good for mind and body. Otherwise, certain indulgences take on a life of their own.

- **Svadhyaya ("study on one's own"):** Deliberating on the sacred texts of Yoga. This practice includes chanting and repeating scriptural writings in order to commit them to memory. But it also applies to all inspirational literature. Through this practice, the student can reach insights that ordinary life blocks from her awareness.

- **Ishvara pranidhana ("submission"):** A concept found in many religious practices, suggesting surrender only to divine providence. Akin to this is faith, surrendering one's thoughts and deeds to one's deity. *Ishvara* is the Sanskrit word for "lord of the universe."

The Schools of Yoga

For a tradition that is as old and comprehensive as Yoga, it naturally follows that there are many approaches. Patanjali's teachings branched off into specialties as time passed. There are approaches to Yoga that can satisfy every spiritual persuasion. Loosely described, they are "schools" of Yoga, although the philosophical approach is mostly what distinguishes them from each other.

All the schools incorporate meditation as a major component of their practice. Each may emphasize the development of a different dimension in the overall physical and psychological makeup of the practitioners, but the goal is essentially the same. They are all grounded in Vedic philosophy, thus sharing the aim of integrating the physical and nonphysical aspects of an individual's life, and attaining a level of consciousness that transcends them.

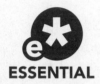

ESSENTIAL

Yoga teachers recognize that any conscious acts that fall into the schools of Yoga are a form of Yoga practice, even though the practitioners may not subscribe to Vedic philosophy or beliefs.

Hatha Yoga

Hatha Yoga is the most commonly recognized form. It primarily combines *asana* ("still posture") and *pranayama* ("breath control"). The body is the primary vehicle in this Yoga practice. Like other meditation approaches that employ physical exercises and discipline, Hatha provides the experience of contrast. The muscles are tensed and then loosened. The body stretches; then it relaxes. This alternation of tension and release is very enlivening, mentally and emotionally. Athletes and sports enthusiasts often attest to this.

Bhakti Yoga

Bhakti (BAK-tee) Yoga is the path of devotion and impersonal love. The "ideal image" is the primary vehicle in this Yoga practice, which may manifest as dedication to a chosen saint or deity, or idealistic service to a cause. Perhaps you have encountered members of the Hare Krishna movement (International Society of Krishna Consciousness or ISKCON), who chant, sing, play music, and proclaim the name of their divinity. Or maybe you have seen Christian charismatics express their devotion to Mother Mary through pilgrimages to holy places and meditative retreats. Such combinations of devotional expression and religious ministry are forms of Bhakti Yoga.

Karma Yoga

In Karma Yoga, "selfless service" is the primary vehicle. Since karma means "action," it is the externalization of moral and spiritual balance in work that expresses this form of Yoga. Most important, it is not work that the individual undertakes to satisfy personal drives or even duty, but a response to whatever the practitioner is called on to address or remedy in his surroundings. The exemplary life and work of Mother Teresa and Dr. Thomas Dooley are examples of Karma Yoga. Healing, social services, and teaching are also forms of Karma Yoga.

FACT

Besides Yoga, karma ("action") may be the most recognized Sanskrit term to Westerners. It suggests negative experience to many, but it really only describes the (present) results of (past) actions. This may pertain to the immediate past, or former lives of an individual. Conditions relating to past actions are considered karmic.

Jnana Yoga

Jnana (j-YAH-nah) Yoga employs processes of mental discrimination and discipline to achieve wisdom. Also regarded as the Yoga of intellects, it promotes insight and inspiration from deep study and contemplation. You do not have to be scholarly to pursue this path. Copying ancient scriptures can lead to enlightenment as much as studying them.

Mantra Yoga

The science of sound is employed in Mantra Yoga to attain harmony, balance, and exalted states of consciousness. This may be achieved through chanting, reciting mantras or "powerful words," and vibrating certain tones and vowels that evoke mystic states of mind. Examples of Mantra Yoga are found in every culture; sacred sounds are used to transport the listener to the realm of spirit.

Tantra Yoga

Tantra Yoga is the Yoga of "ceremony" or "rite," a path of progressive ritual practices designed to raise the life force. A school derived from this path is Kundalini Yoga, which promotes enlightenment through a graduated series of manipulations of all the creative powers in the body: the vital, sexual, and destructive forces. Naturally, most gurus advise strict discipline and training under the guidance of a teacher for practicing this type of Yoga.

ALERT

Becoming aware may not take place in a few minutes, hours, or even days. Modern life rarely accommodates moments for this, because other things demand our awareness, almost all day (and even at night).

Raja Yoga

The "king" of Yogas or "the royal way" emphasizes two stages of Patanjali's Yoga teachings: the mastery of the yamas ("restraints") and the niyamas ("observances"). These guidelines are essential in Raja Yoga, though the remaining six stages of classical Yoga are also included. Both mind and body are the vehicles for this practice.

Ayurveda

An important adjunct to Yoga is the healing path of Ayurveda (*ayur*, "life"; *veda*, "knowledge"). It is an extensive discipline of diagnosis, therapeutics, herbal pharmacology, and preventive medicine. Since it is derived from Yoga philosophy, Ayurveda naturally incorporates meditation as a key practice in healing, and even in the repertoire of training the Ayurvedic physician.

Among the healing approaches in Ayurveda are meditation with mantras and the deep-breathing exercises of Hatha Yoga. Certain asanas from Hatha Yoga are also recommended for strengthening the internal organs and specific functions of the body.

Yoga Starters

If you decide to meditate using one of the Yoga paths, where do you begin? The best way to start is to become aware, beginning with yourself and extending to your immediate surroundings.

You can use a few devices to practice and stay on track with self-awareness, which will lead to meditative experiences. For whichever Yoga path you choose (and you could have one for each day of the week), give yourself just five minutes to do the exercises.

Hatha Yoga

Focus on physical movement. Two optimum times for becoming more aware of your body's functions and rhythms are in the morning upon waking and at night before retiring. In these instances, you are either preparing your body for the daily routine or winding your body down from the day's activities.

FACT

> *Sadhana* ("to complete") is used to describe a process of Yoga practice. One's *sadhana* may, for instance, comprise Yogic postures (*asana*), breathing exercises (*pranayama*), and mental stillness (*dhyana*), or an altogether different set of Yogic practices, depending on the teacher or the practitioner.

Deliberately slow your breathing by taking deeper breaths. Slow down your physical actions and train your eyes on only what you are doing. Choose one daily routine. For example, if you are combing your hair, move deliberately, watching your hand movements and posture. You do not need a mirror because it can be distracting. Think only of what you are doing and nothing else. The next time you perform this action, be as deliberate as before, but change your movements and posture to accomplish the same thing.

Bhakti Yoga

Focus on devotional feeling. Everyone has an ideal person, an individual who personifies all that we strive to become. Honoring that ideal can bring you to an appreciation of those qualities in others and in yourself.

Place a print or photograph (even one cut out of a magazine or newspaper) in a special, elevated area of your personal space. Take the time to examine the image carefully, especially the facial expression. Think of one quality that you most regard, and consider emulating that quality through something you will do in the next twenty-four hours. Place an offering before that image as a reminder of your commitment. It can be a flower, a cone of incense, or your favorite inspirational book.

Karma Yoga

Focus on meaningful activity. Conscious work can be an important meditation, especially if it is something you ordinarily regard as unpleasant.

Choose a necessary task that you must perform by yourself but that you usually put off until the last minute. Examples include laundry, mowing the lawn, or cleaning the birdcage. Plan on doing the chosen task deliberately and with a different attitude. Each time you think or feel how much you want to avoid it, remind yourself that it will be different this time. Move the task to the top of the priority list and proceed. As you are completing the task, think only of the good that will be accomplished when it is done. If it's the laundry, think of the fresh smell of the clothing and the way you will look when wearing it. If it's the lawn, picture the pleasing scene of the finished yard. And if it's the birdcage, recall the pleasant sound of the bird's song.

Jnana Yoga

Focus on clarity of thought. The study of what you regard as important teachings is a means to developing discrimination and mental acuity. Memorizing mathematical formulas can do this, but it rarely applies to practical life.

Choose a saying or proverb that has meaning to you. You may find these in calendars, on websites, or in your personal book collection. For example, "It takes little effort to watch a man carry a heavy load." Write this saying down and leave it in several places, such as your desk, car dashboard, and nightstand. Each time you read the saying, create a variation on the theme. In this case, "It's easy to criticize when you haven't done the work." Make notes of your own variation. Gather all the variations you made under the original saying. You may discover some unique (or strange) insights into your own thinking.

Mantra Yoga

Focus on listening. Some words are pleasing to the ear, even though they may not have any association with people you know or places you've been.

Choose a single word or expression, limiting it to about five syllables (for example, "nightingale"). Recite the word, very slowly for about one minute. Draw out every possible sound from the word, and vibrate those sounds. In this example, the *N*s and the *L* offer good possibilities for humming the sounds. Recite the word for another minute, picking up the pace. Repeat this three more times, each time speeding up the recitation. When you're finished, the word will have evoked sounds, thoughts, and feelings you did not have when you started.

FACT

The earliest writings on Yoga were written in Sanskrit, a language regarded as divine in origin. Many Sanskrit words have no English equivalent; they are very specific to states of meditation and spiritual experience. Though Sanskrit is no longer a living language, terms pertaining to the Yoga tradition are still expressed in the original language.

Tantra Yoga

Focus on habit. We are often unaware of the rituals we create in our life. This is an exercise that can foster an awareness of ourselves, especially under ordinary conditions.

Before starting your daily routine (in the morning or the night before), make a list of what you know that you usually do in the first five minutes. For example: Wake up, pull up the window shade, go to the kitchen and start the coffee, go to the bathroom. Place that list where you will see it immediately. Use as much detail as possible. For instance, if you look out the window after raising the shade and rinse the coffee pot before adding water, make note of it.

At the start of the routine, take the list and follow the steps you have outlined for yourself, as if you are following instructions for the first time. If you notice that you have to do something not on the list, add it as you go. Later, review your list with particular attention to the steps you missed.

Raja Yoga

Focus from the present and future. The integration of body, mind, and spirit is the goal of all Yogas. This goal is not accomplished overnight, but a reminder of it is always a positive effort.

Place yourself in a comfortable position—seated or standing—and face a wide horizon. Looking up at a mountain, across a body of water, or even at the sky is ideal. Take notice of your breathing for the first four minutes. As you do so, picture the air entering your lungs with each inhalation as being pure and colorless. When you exhale, picture the contents of your mind leaving with the air that goes out of your body. Those contents are fragments of color: blue, green, gray, and red.

Recite an affirmation that reminds you of your essential goal for the present. Phrase it as though you have already accomplished that goal. For example, use positive affirmations such as "I am strong for others" or "I am healthy." As you say the words, picture those sounds as being as pure and colorless as the air that enters your body.

CHAPTER 7

Body Dynamics

One reason so many people study Yoga today is that it examines and provides approaches to "tuning" our primary instruments—the body and the mind. With Yoga, we are not asked to ignore the needs and rhythms of physical life but to know them thoroughly and work with them.

The Yoga Universe

You may ask how it's possible to choose one of the many forms of Yoga. Which is easiest or most effective? How can you learn what suits your particular needs and schedule?

Selecting any one of the Yoga paths requires that we first understand some of the fundamentals of Yoga science. The underlying philosophy applies to all the branches in the system. These ideas are not all based in material science, either. The mind and soul are recognized as part of the energy dynamic of life, and Yoga offers a fascinating view of how they work together. This system is both physical and metaphysical. It is a practical guide to progressing through stages of meditation practice.

The Yogi (or Yogini, "female practitioner of Yoga") views the universe as *prakriti*, a reality that possesses three dimensions:

- **Tamas:** The first dimension is the realm of phenomena, the external reality; the objective world, without thought or feeling.
- **Sattva:** The second dimension is the realm of perception. Because it is perceived through our consciousness, it is the subjective world, and is filled with thought and feeling.
- **Rajas:** The third dimension is the realm of pure energy. It is the world of action, neither subjective or objective.

Is this just abstract philosophy? Actually, the Yogi sees the divisions of *prakriti* as a way of categorizing the qualities of mind. We are always in one or more of these dimensions: subjective, objective, and in motion. In meditation, we are involved in discriminating between these states and understanding them. And ultimately, we are seeking to harmonize them, to attain *sat-chit-ananda,* the "state of complete unity," or bliss.

The Yogi also sees the physical body as a miniature universe. Here, it is composed of the *tattwas,* or five elements, which constitute all matter in the objective world. We each possess *agni* (fire), which manifests as sight. *Prithivi* (earth) gives us smell, and *vayu* (air) provides touch. In addition, our bodies possess *jala* (water), which gives the sense of taste, and *akasha* (aether) expressed through hearing.

The Metaphysical Body and the Chakras

In Yoga, the universe and the human body are viewed as separate but mutually dependent entities. How do these two realities interact? Here, Yoga has provided a blueprint for that interaction, and this "invisible anatomy" has become a popular model in Western approaches for meditation, healing, psychology, and even sports.

In this model, the body possesses a number of centers that interchange energy with universal energy. There are seven of these centers, or chakras ("wheels"), within the body, and an eighth surrounds it as an "aura" or energy field. The chakras are located in a line parallel to the spinal cord, and each is centered near one of the vital plexes (which function like junction boxes for the nervous system). In turn, the plexes are associated with one of the major glands in the endocrine system. This is an important consideration in Hatha Yoga, since the practice is concerned with the health and well-being of the body as well as the mind. Meditation is believed to stimulate, among other things, the glands associated with the chakras. Since aging and illness are intrinsically linked to the diminishing of glandular function, this is one reason that consistent practice is regarded as a rejuvenator of internal processes.

The chakras are sometimes depicted as lotus flowers, with different letters or sounds inscribed on each *nadi* ("petal"). These letters or symbols represent the *bija* ("sound syllable") that awakens and stimulates each chakra. A color also corresponds to each chakra, and is associated with the radiant energy released when the chakra is in motion. There is both a power and a limitation of personality influenced by each chakra, as well as a physical sense. The chakras include:

- *Muladhara* (**"Root Center"**): The chakra system begins at the base of the spine with the lotus of four petals. It is located at the sacral plexus and governs the gonads (testes in the male, ovaries in the female). The testes produce testosterone, and the ovaries produce both estrogen and progesterone. The sacred sound is *Lam,* and the color is red. The sense of smell is intensified by this chakra. The root center vitalizes physical strength, and its inverse is fear.
- *Svadhisthana* (**"Center of Self"**): This is the lotus of six petals. It is located at the prostatic plexus and governs the adrenals. These glands release hydrocortisone, which affects metabolism. The sacred sound

is *Vam,* and the color is orange. The sense of taste is intensified by this chakra. The self center vitalizes creativity, and its inverse is indulgence.

- *Manipura* **("Radiant Center"):** This is the lotus of ten petals. It is located in the epigastric plexus and governs the spleen and pancreas. The latter produces insulin, which controls the body's chief energy source, sugar. The sacred sound is *Ram,* and the color is yellow. The sense of sight is intensified by this chakra. The radiant center increases vitality, and its inverse is weakness.

- *Anahata* **("Soundless Center"):** This is the lotus of twelve petals. It is located in the cardiac plexus and governs the thymus. This gland, located behind the breastbone, is important in stimulating cellular immune responses. It also produces cortisone when the body experiences stress. The sacred sound is *Yam* and the color is green. The sense of touch is intensified by this chakra. The soundless center vitalizes compassion, and its inverse is oversensitivity.

- *Vissuddha* **("Pure Center"):** This is the lotus of sixteen petals. It is located in the pulmonary plexus and governs the thyroids and parathyroids. These glands produce a complex of hormones that regulates metabolism, body heat production, and bone growth. The sacred sound is *Ham,* and the color is blue. The sense of sound is intensified by this chakra. The pure center vitalizes courage, and its inverse is instability.

- *Ajna* **("Quiet Center"):** This is the lotus of two petals. It is located in the pharyngeal plexus and governs the pituitary. Regarded as the body's "master gland," the pituitary produces growth hormone and influences the lower glands to secrete. In metaphysical literature, this center is equivalent to the "third eye" of spiritual sight when opened. The sacred sound is *Om* and the color is violet. Thought is intensified by this chakra. The quiet center vitalizes intuition, and its inverse is delusion.

- *Sahasrara* **("Thousand Center"):** This is the lotus of a thousand petals. It is located in the cavernous plexus and governs the pineal. This gland produces melatonin, which governs the body's biorhythms. When opened, this chakra is metaphysically expressed by halos and the royal crowns of monarchs—all are symbols of exalted awareness. Upon taking vows, members of monastic communities will shave the head or wear a tonsure to signify a commitment to opening this center and attaining enlightenment.

How the Chakras Work

How do the chakras work? Two currents of energy flow through the body around a central canal, crossing at the chakras. These currents are the *ida* (negative pole) and the *pingala* (positive pole). The currents originate from the rhythms of the *tattwas*, through changes in the environment, the mind, and the balance of the body itself. The central canal around which the polar energies intertwine is called the *sushumna* and corresponds roughly to the spinal cord. Within it lies the potential force of every individual—the *kundalini*. It is often visualized as a coiled serpent, sleeping at the base of the spine.

The chakras allow the five elements within the body to interact and exchange energy with the three dimensions of the Yogic universe. And although this model of "invisible anatomy" is original to Yoga, it is viewed the same way in the Buddhist tradition.

According to Yoga science, the resulting interchange between these currents and the body is a "vortex" of energy revolving in each chakra. It's just like the rotor of an electric motor that turns when positive and negative charges pass through it.

What purpose do the chakras serve? This is where meditation plays its vital role. If and when the polar energies are flowing freely in the body through the chakras, it becomes possible to "awaken" the *kundalini* force, allowing it to flow upward and penetrate the chakras. As this occurs, certain powers are awakened in both mind and body, some of which are described in the chakra table. Of course, this doesn't happen naturally or at will. The individual's personal development along with Yoga practice will determine its occurrence. Meditation must be used to gain awareness of the energetic nature of the body and allow the chakras to do their work. Then the gradual awakening of the *kundalini* force takes place, and it is harnessed to benefit the practitioner in many ways.

The Energy Environment

Though many of the concepts in Yogic philosophy don't seem grounded in what you've been taught about the "real" world, they do apply to practical matters. One of them, the principle of *akasha,* can be apprehended in everyday situations. For example, have you ever entered a room full of people and felt a welcoming response, even though nothing was said or done directly to you? Or, have you felt hostility or sadness from someone you'd never met before?

FACT

In Greek mythology, Zeus gave Hermes the caduceus, a magical, winged staff with two serpents twined around it. The caduceus brought peace wherever it was used. The caduceus is recognized today as the symbol of the medical profession. The chakra system is identical to the caduceus symbol. The intertwining of the *ida* and *pingala* currents around the *sushumna* canal mirror the path of serpents wound around the caduceus. At the points they intersect, the chakras are found.

In Yoga, this invisible atmosphere is filled with *akasha.* It's the subtle energy the Greek philosophers called the aether, the "glue" of the material world that holds it all together. One of the functions of *akasha* is to transmit the aura fields of nature and people in and around the environment. If you are sensitive to aura fields, you may perceive some of the unspoken thoughts or feelings of those around you.

Hatha Yoga

In the *Yoga Sutras,* Patanjali said, "Asana is that which produces steadiness and bliss." Hatha, the "yoga of effort," is a practice that developed over centuries, stemming from Patanjali's teachings. Its name is derived from Ha ("Sun") and Tha ("Moon"), referring to the union of light and dark, positive and negative forces, within the body and consciousness of the practitioner.

Basically, Hatha Yoga combines the two branches of *asana* ("posture") with *pranayama* ("breath"). Its purpose is to bring the body into equilibrium, so that the flow of energy (*ida* and *pingala*) can be increased and raised consciously and progressively through the chakras.

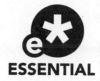

ESSENTIAL

Prana is the breath of life, the life force. It is the first thing to enter our bodies at birth and the last thing to leave when we pass on. When we inhale, we take in *prana*. When we exhale, we expel *apana*, the air that is infused with unfavorable elements to the body.

The central goal of the Yoga *asanas* is the stilling of body and mind. But awakening of the body's natural powers is important, also. That's why the Yogi will visualize the spirit of a Yoga posture and not just perform the physical pose as if something miraculous will automatically happen. One way to view this process is to think of the way the shaman or medicine woman assumes the spirit form of an animal in order to acquire its powers. That way, those powers can be transmitted to the warrior or those who need healing. In Yoga, this same process is undertaken by psychological means. Here, the practitioner emulates the physical and energetic qualities of the posture. That's why most Yoga poses have the names of creatures and forces in the natural world, such as the "grasshopper" and the "mountain."

De-tensing with Breath

Relaxation, or de-tensing, is one of the first steps to preparing the body for meditation in Hatha Yoga. There are several *asanas* for promoting this, but starting with breath is the favored way to proceed.

Choose a posture that allows you to fill your lungs to maximum capacity with *prana*. Sit upright, stand, or lie down—whichever you prefer. Begin with two deep breaths. Remember to take in the *prana* from the ground upward; your stomach should be moving "in-out." On inhaling, pay attention to the sensation of the *prana* filling your lungs. On exhaling, make a conscious effort to empty out all the *apana* in your lungs.

After taking in *prana* for the third time, hold it in, slowly counting one . . . two . . . three . . . . Do not force the *prana* to stay held in your lungs, simply pause as you count from one to five. Then slowly exhale the *apana*, and also make the conscious effort to empty your lungs. Repeat this twice more, so you complete a total of three sets (of three *prana-apanas*).

The Four States of Consciousness

In Yoga philosophy, there are four planes or states of consciousness, known as *avastha* ("states of mind"). In meditation, the practitioner is directed to progress through these stages attentively.

The first state, *jagrat* ("waking consciousness"), is our daily awareness. This includes the five senses, plus thinking and remembering. Before sleeping, we enter a state ("half awake–half asleep") where we are still conscious, but the contents of the mind are receding from our awareness.

The second state is *svapna* ("dreaming"). During sleep, we dream approximately one-third of the time, after entering a preliminary stage of rest and before going into deep sleep. Part of the conscious mind is aware enough to monitor dream activity, and that's why we can recall dream images and experiences.

The third state is *sushupti* ("deep sleep"), which is the state of unconsciousness, in which we are completely unaware of ourselves and what is going on around us. Induced states of unconsciousness, from injury or anesthetics, fall into this realm.

The fourth state is *samadhi* ("divine consciousness"), the beatific state, in which all the senses, the conscious and unconscious mind, meet. It is not altogether rare; it can happen in moments of excitement or rest, when all of our faculties are at complete stillness.

Hatha Yoga Styles

There are several "styles" of Hatha Yoga; most are based on an approach or adaptation of traditional Yoga by a variety of teachers. Many of these styles have reached the West through programs brought by gurus of various Yoga schools in India and Pakistan.

Kripalu Yoga ("compassionate Yoga") emphasizes "focusing inward" by combining Hatha and Raja techniques. Posture, breathing, and meditation are taught in unison to develop self-observation and self-acceptance. Yogi Amrit Desai, founder of the Kripalu Center in Lenox, Massachusetts, developed this style of Yoga in 1970.

Vinyoga ("individual Yoga") emphasizes gradual learning and progressive techniques adapted to the practitioner. It combines *asana* and *pranayama* with mantra and meditation, allowing the student to develop at her own pace. T. K. V. Desikachar, the son of the venerable Yogi Sri Krishnamacharya, developed Vinyoga.

FACT

Pranayama, the other component of Hatha Yoga, promotes deep-breathing exercises that suppress mental restlessness and enhance both control and relaxation, physically and mentally. The practice of *pranayama* is also the practice of regulating the life force, because breath is essential to enhancing and prolonging life.

Ashtang Yoga ("eightfold Yoga") refers to the original eight limbs of Yoga practice. This style emphasizes action and awareness. The aim is to develop "internal heat" by focusing on muscular strength and "body locks," combining progressive sets of asanas with breathing techniques. Developed by K. Pattabhi Jois in the 1990s, it quickly acquired the name "power Yoga" because of its emphasis on athletic endurance.

Awakening: The Alternating Breath

This breathing exercise is taught in nearly all Yoga schools and styles as an "awakening" technique to vitalize both body and mind. Often used as a prelude to meditation, its Sanskrit name is Anulom Viloma. With it, you also place your active hand in a gesture known as the Vishnu Mudra ("sign of preservation"). The index and middle fingers are tucked into the palm of the hand, leaving the thumb, third finger, and little finger open. You will be using the thumb to close the right nostril, and the third and little fingers to close the left nostril. The steps of the exercise are as follows:

1. Start with an upright spine. Place your active hand in the Vishnu Mudra.
2. Close the right nostril with the thumb, inhale deeply through the left nostril.
3. Close both nostrils, hold in your breath to the count of eight.

4. Release the right nostril; exhale slowly.
5. Keeping the left nostril closed, inhale deeply through the right nostril.
6. Close both nostrils; hold in your breath to the count of eight.
7. Release left nostril; exhale slowly.
8. These steps constitute one round of Anulom Viloma, which may be practiced in eight rounds.

The Human Body: A Work of Art

Every aspect of Hatha Yoga practice—*asana* and *pranayama*—begins with the consideration of what is natural for the body's anatomy. What is natural? Let's take a look at some of the basics that apply to a healthy Hatha Yoga program.

Spine

The spinal cord is our "pillar of life." It supports the entire skeletal structure and is comprised of twenty-four separate, flexible vertebrae and an additional nine that are fused together at the base of the spine. This creates four regions: the sacral (at the base of the spine), the lumbar (lower back), the thoracic (upper back), and the cervical (neck). Between the flexible vertebrae are discs of tough, connective tissue that absorb weight and shock while the spine is at rest and in motion. For the spine to be healthy, it should have three natural curves that form an *S* shape:

- **Cervical curve:** the concave curve in the neck
- **Thoracic curve:** the convex curve in the back
- **Lumbar curve:** the concave curve in the lower back

Posture

Good posture is more than keeping your spine upright. When standing, your back should be straight enough to feel as though a string hanging from the ceiling would pass down through your head to the floor. One way to test this is to back up against a wall. The length of your spine should be as close to the wall as possible. If it's not, move your feet forward, away from the wall, and slide down a few inches. Then slowly back up and against the wall in tiny steps. Your head should not be tilted; the chin should be slightly raised.

When sitting in a chair, the entire line of your spine should touch the back support. Always remember to position your spine backward and not forward. Once again, your head should not be tilted, with chin slightly raised.

When sitting unsupported, as in meditation, avoid slouching or straining. If you are unused to sitting unsupported, try to acclimate your back by starting with a support in your lumbar curve. Sit against a flat surface, like a wall, and place a rolled-up towel or small, round pillow in the lumbar curve as you lean back.

Nerves and Muscles

The spinal cord is also a channel for the nervous system, which extends from the brain to every limb and organ. The nervous system provides the "electricity" that stimulates the muscles to work and the organs to operate. In turn, the muscles do the work, expanding and contracting so the body can move.

ALERT

Nothing should interfere with the "electric" flow through the complex network of nerves and muscles. That's why shoes, belts, and any restrictive clothing must be avoided in Yoga practice.

Balance

Everyone has an individual point of balance based on height, weight, and body type. Finding your balance may take some time, but it is worth the effort in order to gain the maximum benefit of meditation. After all, if your body is working against the postures and exercises of meditation, you will feel uncomfortable and want to give up the practice.

The keys to finding balance are as follows:

- Avoid straining in any posture.
- Allow breathing to oxygenate the nerves and muscles.
- Build your meditation sessions by graduating time, the number of breathing exercises, and the variation of body postures (*asanas*).

Yoga Asana: The Half Locust and Full Locust

The Half Locust exercise is performed prone, facedown. It strengthens the sacral region and tones the internal organs. It is an excellent prelude to a meditation session.

Lie facedown on a flat surface with your chin touching the floor and your legs extended. Your ankles should be close together; toes pointed outward. Your arms may be at your sides with palms flat on the floor, or under your body with clenched fists. Inhale on raising one leg; exhale on lowering. Focus on slowly stretching the leg as it is raised. Start with one side; follow with the other. Take your time. Raise the leg as high as possible without straining. You can count from one to ten if you want.

Do not bend your legs while they are being raised and avoid tensing the leg and calf muscles. Do not turn or twist the spine at any time.

The Full Locust is a continuation of the Half Locust. Stay in the prone position, facedown with your chin touching the floor and your legs extended. Move your arms under your body, either clenched in fists or grasping the thighs. Inhale, pressing your legs together and stretching them from the toes outward. Raise your legs together while inhaling. Silently count from one to ten. Lower your legs together while exhaling.

CHAPTER 8

The Way of the Senses

Body and mind will always be involved in the practice of meditation. But there is another important dimension of consciousness that we often overlook, much to our detriment. The five senses are important tools for understanding and self-awareness. Without them, our world would be colorless indeed.

The Tantric Tradition

Experiments done in sensory deprivation, in which a person is suspended in a water tank and isolated from sights and sounds of the outside world for an extended period, are revealing. With only the inner world to respond to and with no outer stimuli, subjects suffered from panic and depression. These results tell us that we need sensory experience to be mentally healthy.

FACT

Tantra ("rite" or "prescription") follows the scheme of energy dynamics in the body as taught in traditional Yoga. It teaches a psychospiritual path that harnesses and employs physical powers to reach enlightenment. Compared to many of the ascetic practices of Yoga that constrain the senses and discipline the mind, Tantric Yoga is a system that actually exploits those dimensions of experience.

Several branches of Yoga address just this need. They offer techniques for developing and refining the senses, enabling them to operate optimally. These branches of Yoga also involve unique forms of meditative experience that bring us closer to our inner powers.

The Union of Opposites

One characteristic of Tantric belief is that all life comes into being through the union of the *atman* (Spirit) and the *Shakti* (Nature). This applies to everything—from the universe, filled with galaxies and stars, to human beings and all the life forms on earth. The effort in Yoga is directed toward bringing about a union between the individual *atman* (the self) and the individual Shakti (the *kundalini* force in the body).

This is often depicted in Tantric art and iconography as divine couples in active embrace. Such images are used for meditation on the mystery and fulfillment of "joining opposites" within the meditator, and between the meditator and the universe. Not only is there plenty of sexual imagery in this system, there are also some branches of Tantrism that actually employ sexual embrace, either literally or symbolically, to accomplish this goal. They may be intended to advance only the practitioner in harnessing the powers of body and mind, or they may be meant to bring both partners to a level of *samadhi* ("divine rapture"). The symbolism of the Tantric universe is the means used in meditation. This symbolism has many layers of meaning; it applies to psychological states, physical experience, involvement with a partner, and the practitioner's relationship to external reality.

Meditation During Sex

Yes, this is regarded as a legitimate approach to refining awareness and experiencing physical harmony. Some Tantric methods (although certainly not all) espouse the practice of meditation before, during, and after sexual intimacy. How is this done?

In Yoga, the fundamental approach to maximizing the body's capacity for vitality is *pranayama*. This is no different in Tantric practice. The performance of breathing exercises in unison and the exchange of *prana* by the couple forms part of this Tantric practice.

As in Yoga, certain *asanas* are conducive to enhancing sensitivity and endurance. The couple may employ specific postures to promote this. For example, facing each other in the sitting lotus position, a meditation may be directed to combine the energies between the individual chakras of the couple.

A perfectly choreographed set of Tantric rites is usually performed to heighten the awareness of the couple. For example, the traditional five elements are absorbed in a sacred meal of *madya* (wine), *mansa* (meat), *matsya* (fish), *mudra* (gestures and grain), and *maithuna* (sexual intercourse). These ingredients are taken in by the couple with great deliberation and awareness in order to absorb the maximum amount of life force.

The Tantric school of Yoga that elevates sexual experience in meditation practice is not the same Tantrism practiced in some schools of Buddhism. The Vajrayana branch of Tibetan Buddhism is considered Tantric, as is the Shingon branch of Buddhism in Japan. However, the concept of the union of opposites is important in all Tantric writings and practices. It is an idea that is mirrored in many important meditation techniques for balancing body and mind.

A Tantric Breath

Tantric breath is a way of consciously uniting the energy paths in the body. In Yoga science, the Moon (*ida*, the passive or negative) governs the left side of the body while the Sun (*pingala*, the active or positive) governs the right side. In healing, this concept is applied to drawing in cool air (the left) or warm air (the right) for desired conditions.

In an upright posture, place the right hand index and middle fingers against the right nostril. Take in *prana* slowly and deliberately through the left nostril, then exhale. Direct your attention to the left side of the body (ida), becoming vitalized by the *prana*.

ESSENTIAL

A couple may perform the Tantric breath together. Facing each other, perform the exercise with each one breathing from the opposite side of the other, like a mirror image.

The next breath will be taken in from the right nostril, with the left hand index and middle fingers against the left nostril. Once again, take in *prana* slowly and deliberately; then exhale. Direct your attention to the right side of the body (*pingala*), becoming vitalized by the *prana*. You may start with three sets of breathing (each set equals both sides).

Once completed, rest your hands on your knees or lap, and repeat the exercise the same number of times, this time without closing the nostrils. Direct your attention, as before, to each side becoming vitalized by the *prana*.

Sense Meditations

One important view that the Tantric approach offers is the mindful use of the senses. Although we look and listen every day, we often do not see or hear what is important to our well-being. Meditation that employs the senses to focus is not only useful; it allows us to become aware of things that can make a positive difference in our lives. The following sections cover some sense meditations that will help you develop this awareness.

Seeing

In our modern world, we are subjected to millions of visual images on a daily basis. Of course, in order to influence the buying public's thinking, marketers use repetition to exploit this fact. This repetition may not be altogether harmful, but it does crowd out images that can be helpful when the need arises. How do you counter the problem? Meditate on helpful images.

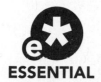

ESSENTIAL

Whenever you encounter a moment of visual fatigue, close your eyes and mentally evoke the image you practiced in meditation. You can change images whenever you find pleasing or soothing alternatives. You can also add to your "archive," using different images for different situations.

Start with a picture, drawing, or representation of something you really enjoy. Place it in front of your meditation sitting area, so you can see all the details. Focus your attention on this image. Take your time looking at its color. Notice how the light around it affects the shade, shadow, and depth of the color. Now close your eyes and see those same details. Take your time to evoke in your mind all that you saw with your eyes opened. Open your eyes to see if the visual image is the same as the mental image. If you notice a difference, do the exercise once more.

Hearing

Noise is another problem we deal with in modern life. There are the insistent electronic sounds from computers, the microwave oven, and cell phones. Then there's traffic, television, and those annoying intercom announcements while shopping. Is it possible to have absolute quiet?

Actually, complete absence of sound is unnatural and can trigger negative episodes. But how much is too much? That is up to the individual.

Start your meditation session when you are certain you will not be interrupted. In your most comfortable meditation posture, begin with closed eyes. Start to listen. Begin with the farthest sounds you can identify. For example, if you hear water running from a faucet down the hallway, listen to it, to the exclusion of all else. The goal is to hear only the running faucet, nothing else. When that takes place, go to the next sound that presents itself, nearer to you. For example, if you hear the wind blowing against the window of the room you're in, listen to it, to the exclusion of all else. Use the same degree of attention as before.

FACT

Many indigenous people, from Polynesian canoe families to the Amazonian forest tribes, have developed an extremely acute sense of hearing. Their survival depends on it, and they also use the skill to entertain and communicate.

You will next listen to an even closer sound. For example, the sound of the cushion you are sitting on, moving in unison with your breath or the motion of your body. Listen to this sound as attentively as you listened to the others. When you begin with the sounds farthest away and move toward those nearest to you, perhaps even getting to the sounds of your breath and heartbeat, you have completed the exercise.

When you are dealing with unpleasant sounds outside of meditation, use this practice to listen to other sounds that will neutralize those you do not wish to hear.

Touching

The sense of touch conveys a great deal of information that we might otherwise miss by just looking and listening. According to Yoga science, the sense of touch leads to understanding in a manner that regular learning cannot fulfill.

Those who work with clay and other plastic media attest to the meditative experience they provide. Here, you're not only focused on transferring a mental image to a physical embodiment. The act of working with the material itself is a meditation, because you notice all of the nuances of movement. The subtle flow of action and reaction become apparent, and "noticing" attains more clarity. Here's a meditative approach: Look for a good exercise medium to develop your sense of touch. This could be Play-Doh, Silly Putty, or any of the soft, therapeutic exercise balls sold in sports equipment stores. All you need is a supple, pliable medium that fits your hand and maintains its original shape or returns to it.

In your most comfortable meditation posture, begin with opened eyes. It is best to start with the hand that you do not use normally. For example, if you are right-handed, start with your left hand, and vice versa.

Work the plastic material slowly. Begin by pressing it and noticing the reaction of the material (you could use your sense of hearing, too). Give this two minutes, maximum. While you are working the material, take notice of its response to your pressing, squeezing, and turning.

Remember that you are not testing your memory, but transferring the visual image to a mental image with as much detail as possible. Think of your eyes as a scanning device, copying the complete picture to your inner meditation archive.

Remember that this is not an artistic exercise to "create something." Rather, it is a way of using your sense of touch to monitor the response of the material to your efforts.

When you stop, close your eyes. Take notice of the sensations in your hand. Start from the wrist; move outward toward the palm. From the palm, move toward each finger, in turn. With each finger, move from the base to the tip. Here, you are monitoring the response of your hand to both the material and the efforts you made while working with the material.

FACT

Some people are more visual than sensual; their understanding is more easily achieved through seeing than by touching. In fact, some research says that women are more "touchy-feely" than men, while men are more stimulated by images than sensations. But this may be more of a cultural phenomenon than one of gender.

Open your eyes, and now practice this with your other hand (if you started with the left, go to the right). It is quite revealing to notice how this hand may be more or less sensitive than the one you started with. You could continue in future meditation sessions with efforts to equalize the degree of sensitivity in both hands.

Mandala, Mantra, and Mudra

These words are specialized, meditative approaches to seeing, hearing, and touching. The Tantric school of Yoga makes great use of these devices to aid in focusing attention and transforming the meditative state from one level to another. Mandala uses image; mantra employs sound; and mudra engages through gesture. As is the ritual nature of Tantra, these devices are symbolic ways to reach and emulate exalted states of consciousness. We will explore the fascinating realms of mandala imagery and mantra sounds later. For now we'll look at the practice of mudra, which is a beneficial way to focus your physical presence in the practice of meditation.

Mudra ("sign" or "gesture") is a way of linking action with a state of mind. You are undoubtedly familiar with the gesture of praying, with upright hands folded together at the chest. If you see someone in this pose, you assume that person is praying. You make that assumption because it is an example of a gesture that has universal recognition. So it is with mudra. Practitioners of Yoga and Buddhist meditation use similar mudras, since the latter tradition arose from the former. You may have seen pictures of Yogis in meditation, or a seated Buddha in a shrine. Notice the hand gestures of these images, because they convey profound meaning to the meditator.

For meditation, the use of mudras that have time-honored significance can promote certain states of mind and feeling. Anjali mudra is the world-recognized gesture of prayer. Upright hands are folded at the chest level, and the thumbs are pressed against the sternum. In cultures where it is used in greeting others, it conveys the state of "sameness" and honoring the other.

Dhyani mudra is the gesture of meditation. With both hands open, relaxed, and facing upward, the right is "cupped" in the left at the level of the waist. If sitting, the hands are rested in this position in the lap. The tips of the thumbs may be touching. This represents receptivity and stillness.

Vitarka mudra is the gesture of the Buddha. The thumb and index fingers are curled in a circle and touching each other, while the remaining fingers are relaxed together. In sitting meditation, the hands may assume this gesture while resting on the knees or thighs. The circle evokes calm; the extended fingers represent harmony.

Kundalini Yoga

For centuries, certain techniques in Yoga practice were reserved for only the most advanced practitioners. As with Tantra Yoga, these were viewed as either too powerful or, depending on the moral climate of the times, too daring for social acceptance.

One of these approaches is Kundalini Yoga. Derived from Tantric practice, it aims to awaken the latent forces in the body through specific Yogic exercises. Of rather modern origin, the practice is more comprehensive or "holistic" than the ancient version. Kundalini emphasizes diet, meditation, and personal involvement with the outer world through service. The Indian master Swami Vishnu Shivananda, a physician and Yoga scholar, first introduced kundalini to the West in 1935.

FACT

One of the first to actively teach Kundalini Yoga practice in the West was Yogi Bhajan. Born in Pakistan of Sikh parentage, he came to the United States in 1969 to teach Yoga to a growing number of spiritual seekers. Followers don't have to be "religious" to reap the rewards of his comprehensive program of meditation, Yoga, and guidance in the vegetarian lifestyle.

As the name implies, the aim of this practice is the raising of the *kundalini* force through meditative practice. It's also known as the "serpent power" of the body because of its serpentine imagery and flow (remember the caduceus). As it rises in the body during meditation, the *kundalini* penetrates the chakras and awakens their energies. The practitioner focuses inwardly on this activity, continuing upward. The force then unites with Shiva in the crown chakra, where "divine union" is achieved.

Bhakti Yoga

The philosophy of Yoga allows for all types of personalities and expressions. Among its many byways, there is room for the intellectual, the sensualist, and the devotional types. It is the last that accounts for some of the more admirable—and sometimes quite perplexing—approaches in meditation. Bhakti Yoga is a way to develop exalted awareness through devotional activity. But, we might wonder, how can a person attain stillness while doing this?

Now we enter into the realm of meditative practice that is all about doing, and that is truly what most of meditation is about. Yes, there are moments of stillness, observation, and awareness. But there will also be a time for applying the focus and insight attained in these acts through action in the outer world, "reality." It is inevitable, and it often happens naturally. Focus and insight can be applied through love, devotion, and nondiscriminatory service to what is around us.

Meditation on Compassion

Compassion, one of the innate human qualities, is awakened in meditation. You may not be expecting this, but an awareness of the feelings and thoughts of those around you increases as your awareness of yourself grows. Obviously, one person cannot alleviate the suffering of the world, but responding with compassion when you are faced with suffering can make your life richer and more meaningful.

FACT

There are many examples of Bhakti Yoga in the everyday world. The inspirational work of Mother Teresa is one of them. Through devotion to the ideal of Christ's dictate to alleviate the suffering of others, she put philosophy into a lifetime practice. Other religious and historical figures have performed in the same way throughout history, in many places and circumstances.

If you enter a meditation session with some concerns about the problems around you, a compassionate meditation may be called for. The one presented here is adapted from Harry Palmer's book *Resurfacing*. You can practice it whenever you find yourself at odds with either the environment or those around you. And you may want to rephrase any of it to be more meaningful to the situation. Whatever the case, the idea is to encourage an overall sense of understanding and compassion in your outlook on everyone and everything.

Find a person who may embody the concerns you have, and direct your thoughts to that person. Avoid looking at that person so as not to draw attention. With your mental focus on the image of the person, say to yourself:

Just like me, this person is seeking some happiness in his life. Just like me, this person is trying to avoid suffering in his life. [Maintain your mental focus.] Just like me, this person has known sadness, loneliness, and despair. Just like me, this person is seeking to fill his needs. Just like me, this person is learning about life.

A Bhakti Yoga Luminary

Swami Bhaktivedanta Prabhupada (1896–1977) founded the Hare Krishna movement in 1966, known in the West as the International Society for Krishna Consciousness (ISKCON). Placing the life of Krishna, the legendary incarnation of the deity Vishnu, as the divine ideal, the practitioner attains union with divine consciousness. Krishna was chosen because it is believed that in the Kali Yuga, the dark age in which we live, the incarnation of divine light comes from this image. Besides serving this image through devoted effort, the chanting of the Maha Mantra ("great chant") banishes negative forces and evokes the positive influence of divinity.

QUOTE

"Strive to practice the presence."

—Patanjali, *The Yoga Sutras*

Though some may judge this practice to be nonsensical and mindless, the practice of repeating divine names is as old as the human race. It is closely associated with prayer, and is always found in some form when encountering devoted action. Its purposes are diverse:

- To infuse the mind with divine consciousness
- To banish the influences of materialism
- To focus attention on devoted thought and feeling

The Maha Mantra is very simple, and you may have heard it before. The recordings of former Beatle George Harrison are infused with some of the chant. Here, the name of Krishna is spoken, along with the name of Rama, one of the heroic incarnations of Vishnu. The word *hare* means "hail," and it suggests the awakening or evocation of the divine presence: "Hare Krishna, Hare Krishna, Krishna, Krishna, Hare, Hare. Hare Rama, Hare Rama, Rama, Rama, Hare, Hare."

Raja Yoga

Though all Yogas emphasize meditation, Raja Yoga is viewed as the culmination of all. Here, the process emphasizes the freeing of the mind from all influences brought by the senses. Since the senses are part of the realm of *maya* (illusion), the mind cannot be liberated through meditation until it is detached from the sensations of the physical needs, emotions, and beliefs.

Raja Yoga employs *hatha* techniques to relax the body and train breathing, but its primary approach is harnessing the powers of the mind. Raja also espouses a rather ascetic approach, eliminating attachment of the senses one by one. These feats have been recorded under laboratory conditions.

To pursue Raja Yoga is to follow and master the eight-step protocol of Yogic practice outlined by Patanjali. Once again, the eight steps include:

- *Yama* (restraints)
- *Niyama* (purifications)
- *Asana* (posture)
- *Pranayama* (breath)
- *Pratyahara* (withdrawal)
- *Dharana* (concentration)
- *Dhyana* (meditation)
- *Samadhi* (absorption)

A Yogi Tea Break

After a meditation session, tea offers a stimulating transition to the world of work and play. The ingredients in this Yogi tea are the traditional spices used in Indian cooking. They are an excellent way to allow the body to perspire in the hot climate while having a much-needed refreshment. Here's a recipe for two cups.

Yogi Tea
1 teaspoon black tea (Ceylon, Darjeeling, or gunpowder)
4 black peppercorns or one sprinkle of coarse black pepper
4 cardamom seedpods (squeeze between your fingers to open) or one sprinkle of cardamom powder
2 cloves or one sprinkle of clove powder
1 stick of cinnamon or one sprinkle of cinnamon powder
1½ cups cold water
½ cup milk (regular or low fat)

Add the tea and all spices to the water in a small pan and bring it to a boil. Allow it to simmer; then add the milk. When it comes to a rolling simmer, remove the tea from the stove and strain it into a cup. You can float the cardamom seeds in the teacup to enjoy their fragrance as you sip the tea.

Tea drinking in cultures where meditation is commonly practiced is also a time-honored form of meditation. This is because some of the exercises in concentration and physical stamina are viewed as work, albeit of a spiritual nature. Still, the tea break is an accepted way for the meditator to pause and refresh, while maintaining the meditative atmosphere.

CHAPTER 9

Mind Dynamics

In Western society, we spend eight years in elementary and middle school, four in high school, and four or more years pursuing higher education. Then, we are supposed to be fully prepared to use our knowledge to earn a living and participate socially and politically in the world. But most likely, few people truly believe they possess the full capability to do these things.

The Buddhist Tradition

Much of the insecurity and self-doubt that many experience at work and in relationships comes from a lack of education about the inner life. The world of the mind and the role of emotions are relegated to special studies in psychology and sociology but rarely to practical training.

Knowing and experiencing the full dimension of mind is a science that can be learned without experts or special education. After all, it is your mind, isn't it? You will need to dedicate a certain amount of time to this, of course. But you more than anyone else are the best qualified to unlock and explore the potential you possess.

Buddhism, like Yoga, is an integrated system of belief, practice, and wide cultural traditions. Over centuries of development, Buddhist teachings include philosophy, religious practice, medicine, and a repository of language and customs. Today there are 250 million followers of Buddhism, mostly in Asia. However, interest in this tradition has grown since its introduction to the West in the nineteenth century, and about 250,000 people now practice some form of Buddhism in the West.

FACT

A *bikshu* is a Buddhist monk who seeks food and shelter by wandering. He may live periodically in the monastery, but the aim is to follow the Buddha's example of preaching the dharma.

While Buddhism is regarded as one of the world's great religions, most practitioners regard it neither as a religion nor as a philosophy. Rather, it is viewed as a body of approaches to individual enlightenment using the life and teachings of the Buddha as guideposts. There are hundreds of "schools" of Buddhist thought, and each offers a valid approach to the goal of enlightenment. While there has been some disagreement about which approaches are closer to the Buddha's teachings or intentions, there is much overall agreement. Each school of Buddhist thought arose from the social and environmental issues of the time. As a result, there are a number of approaches for the modern seeker to explore.

Buddhism's Adaptability

The adaptability of Buddhism over the ages has contributed to its endurance and prominence in many countries. In the West, it has been met with tremendous interest. Many of the traditional schools of Buddhism have large followings in North American and European communities. This has prompted greater adaptation, so much so that secular approaches derived from Buddhist teachings have arisen in recent times. There are meditation programs for health and psychological clarity, and even mediation training for social and cultural disputes.

Buddhism continues to have considerable influence on the cultures that have absorbed it. The qualities of serenity and patience, for example, are highly valued in Buddhist societies far more than sensation and willpower. This is because Buddhism emphasizes the transmutation of raw force into refined energy. Meditation is seen as the primary means to achieve this.

Other characteristics of Buddhist culture include respect for those who are spiritually accomplished, and the elders in society. There is a high regard for spiritual tradition, which is more important than fads or trends. That is one reason so many Westerners have turned to Buddhist philosophy and practices, seeing those features as missing in modern life.

What Is a Buddha?

The term Buddha is generic, derived from the Sanskrit *budh,* meaning "to awaken or perceive." Buddha is used to denote a person who is awakened or illuminated, who has attained the status of a fully realized human being. By achieving this status, a practitioner eliminates suffering in her life. But the Buddhist goal does not stop there. Understanding the causes of suffering and discovering a personal approach to eliminating them is fundamental to several Buddhist practices.

Another associated concept is the bodhisattva, an individual who is the Buddhist equivalent to a Christian saint, one who is but a few steps from attaining Buddhahood. The term is also used to describe individuals who have achieved illumination but remain in earthly life to alleviate the suffering of their fellow human beings. One of the best-known bodhisattvas is Avalokitesvara, the Buddha of compassion. He periodically returns to the world to alleviate the ills of humanity and is believed by the Tibetans to incarnate, or return to the physical world, in the body of the Dalai Lamas.

Who Was the Buddha?

In 1976, archeologists unearthed the site of Kapilavastu, a city established 3,000 years ago. Located nearly ten miles from Lumbini, Nepal, it is, according to tradition, the city of the historical Buddha's birth.

The man we know as the Buddha was born here as Siddhartha in 563 B.C.E. to the royal house of the Gautama clan of the Nepalese Sakya (SHAK-yah) tribe. Although he spent his youth as a prince in sheltered circumstances, he sought answers to the problems of life in the world outside the palace. In pursuit of this, he abandoned his life of luxury and at age twenty-nine assumed the identity of a *sannyasin,* an itinerant holy man.

In the first six years, Siddhartha subjected himself to the ascetic practices of the *sannyasins* of his time and gradually gathered a group around him. He and his companions believed that by mortifying the flesh one could become liberated from it, and meditation was one means of maintaining this belief. But he realized the inadequacy of this approach, and retreated to meditation under a sacred fig tree, the legendary Bodh-Gaya. It was here, while sitting in a lotus position in meditation, that Sakyamuni ("the wise man of the Sakya tribe") attained *bodhi* ("enlightenment").

The Buddha did not begin his mission of teaching for some years, believing that what he discovered could not be understood by most. However, he did embark on an extensive journey of public ministry after he gave his first sermon in the Deer Park, near Benares, India. In this sermon, he outlined the Four Noble Truths, which form the essential doctrine of Buddhism.

According to tradition, Siddhartha reached enlightenment in four stages. As he sat in deep meditation under the fig tree, Mara, the demon of illusion, approached him. To prevent Siddhartha from reaching his goal, Mara sent three of his confederates: Flurry, Gaiety, and Sullen Pride. But they failed to deter Siddhartha from his goal. Next, three more obstacles were sent: Thirst, Discontent, and Delight. They also failed to break their victim.

Buddhist chronicles, like the parables of the New Testament and the wisdom stories of Native Americans, convey great truths disguised in narratives. The obstacles sent to Siddhartha represent the attitudes and desires that prevent us from approaching our innate wisdom. The protagonist's victory, however, is a potential victory for us as well. That is why such stories can serve as guideposts along the road to enlightenment.

QUOTE

"If the Buddha is to be called a savior at all, it is only in the sense that he discovered and showed the path to liberation, Nirvana. But we must tread the path ourselves."

—Ven. Dr. W. Rahula

After dispelling these obstacles, Siddhartha reached the first stage of enlightenment. In it, he was able to see all of his former lives, and he came to understand the cycle of rebirth. He also understood the suffering brought by rebirth and its causes. In the second stage, he saw through all the illusions that veil true reality and acquired the "heavenly eye." In the third stage of enlightenment, Siddhartha came to understand the true nature of existence, but there is no instruction for this. It is up to the Buddhist practitioner to discover this individually. In the fourth stage, Siddhartha entered the state of enlightenment and became a Buddha. Once again, only the practitioner can know and experience the meaning of this achievement.

One of the great accomplishments of the Buddha's teaching was the inclusion of women and all classes of people in the pursuit of enlightenment. Formerly, Hindu society was firmly entrenched in a caste system, in which only the higher classes could engage in spiritual pursuits. The Buddha saw that all sentient beings (those who possess senses) are capable of enlightenment. This approach of "spiritual democracy" is well understood to this day in all forms of Buddhist teaching and practice.

The Four Noble Truths

The Buddha's first doctrine, taught after he attained enlightenment, became the basis for all Buddhist philosophy. In it, he describes the origins and the outcome of human existence. These precepts are not meant to discourage or denigrate human experience; rather, they are meant to offer insight into ways of transforming it toward a supreme goal.

The first noble truth states that suffering is the heritage of all sentient beings. Birth, pain, old age, and death are the realities that all must experience; these realities are inescapable. Moreover, they are impermanent, although all beings are subject to their repetition according to their own karma.

The second noble truth is that desire and ignorance bring about the endless cycle of suffering. These conditions produce karmic patterns, which perpetuate the cycle of rebirth.

The third noble truth speaks of the denial of the self (the false identity). This denial can overcome the pain of impermanence and allow the practitioner to reach liberation from the cycle of rebirth.

The fourth noble truth articulates the actions that may eliminate the causes of suffering, also known as the Eightfold Path. The actions include right view (or attitude), right thought, right speech, right action, right livelihood, right effort, right mindfulness, and right concentration. Together they promote the development of the three fundamentals: morality, concentration, and wisdom.

FACT

One of the symbols you will encounter repeatedly in Buddhist art is the *Dharmachakra* ("wheel of the law"). It is an eight-spoke wheel that represents the eightfold path to liberation. It is in perpetual motion, spreading the Buddha's teachings through time and space. It is often seen with accompanying deities, who act as guardians of the dharma.

The Eightfold Path is the key to personal transformation on the Buddhist path. Each component is an effort that leads to enlightenment. However, the student does not approach it in a linear way, but holistically. All eight approaches must be active in the practitioner's mind and action. In meditative practice, these components can be seeds for contemplation, direction, and action in a person's life.

The combined efforts of an individual toward realizing the Four Noble Truths and practicing the Eightfold Path lead to nirvana. This is the supreme goal of all Buddhist practice.

The Schools of Buddhism

The Buddha left worldly life at age eighty. After his passing in 483 B.C.E., his close followers met and began the task of recording his teachings and organizing a monastic rule for future followers. As a result, there are now a variety of schools, or branches, of Buddhism. Each may be seen as a side of the many-faceted jewel of Buddhist thought; unlike other religions, there is a conspicuous absence of theological dispute among Buddhist sects. They are mostly in agreement, only emphasizing different areas of the Buddha's teaching.

Mahayana

Mayahana ("great vehicle") is predominant in the northern countries of Asia including China, Japan, and Vietnam. In 100 B.C.E. Buddhism branched into two schools: the Mahayana and the Theravada, the latter adhering strictly to the early Buddhist scriptures.

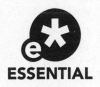

ESSENTIAL

Nirvana ("liberation" and "extinction") is the stage of enlightenment where illumination is achieved and the individual life merges with the universal "cause." In this sense, individual identity becomes "extinct." This is the goal of all Buddhist practice.

There are a number of important branches on the Mahayana tree, each possessing several unique approaches to meditation. One well-known branch is Zen, which developed over the centuries in Japan. It features a combination of ascetic practice, meditation, and introspection exercises.

Theravada

Theravada ("tradition of the elders") is the oldest form of Buddhism, almost exclusive to the island of Sri Lanka and dominating the southern countries of Asia including Laos and Thailand.

Vajrayana

Vajrayana ("vehicle of the diamond") is the Tantric school of Buddhism, which grew out of the Mahayana branch. It is predominant in northwestern Asia including Nepal, Tibet, and Mongolia.

Vajrayana Buddhism was established in eighth century Tibet by the legendary guru, Padmasambhava. Masters of Tantra are called *siddhas,* the "faultless ones." Tantric Buddhism emphasizes the image or appearance of devotional figures, such as the Buddha, bodhisattvas, and both protective and adversarial demons. Ritual, mantra (sound), and mudra (gesture) are incorporated in the practice of meditation. The concept of *shunyata* ("emptiness") is central to this school, and it can be approached through either ascetic practices or full engagement of the senses—there is much adaptation to the outside world in this philosophy. Visualization and imagination are vital meditation tools of this school.

The Three Jewels of Buddhism

All Buddhist communities and organizations support three jewels, or objectives. They constitute the goals and activities of Buddhist practice. All three are equally important, and the practitioner is expected to give time and effort to each equally.

Buddha ("Enlightened One")

Honoring the historical Buddha brings merit but only if his teachings become an active part of the practitioner's life. The Buddha's life is viewed as a prototype of spiritual progress that applies to every life. Enlightened beings existed before the Buddha, and many more have come and will continue to enter the "wheel of life" to aid others in attaining enlightenment. Thus, seeking and cultivating the Buddha nature in oneself and others is a goal of Buddhist practice.

Dharma ("Carrying")

This is the expression of universal truth, referring to the work or teachings of the Buddha. It includes ethics, rules and guidelines of the tradition, and the work the practitioner performs individually to cultivate and spread Buddhist ideas. Seeking and understanding one's own dharma is also important spiritual work. To discover our purpose in life and fulfill it is one of the great merits in Buddhism.

FACT

The principal scriptures were originally recorded in the ancient languages of India: Pali and Sanskrit. As time passed, they were translated into Chinese, Tibetan, and Japanese. Most Buddhist terms are derived from Vedic tradition, so they pertain to ideas in both Yoga and Buddhism.

Sangha ("Community")

Initially referring to the monastic body to which the Buddhist student belongs, the *sangha* also applies to the worldwide family of Buddhism, including those who follow the precepts of the Buddha. Supporting the *sangha* brings merit to the practitioner. This also means tolerating and finding common ground with other Buddhist traditions.

Eliminating Suffering

In Buddhist teaching, three problems in life, called the "three poisons," are identified as the cause of all suffering. They are anger (or ill will), greed (or covetousness), and folly (delusion or stupidity). The goal of spiritual practice is to transmute anger into serenity, greed into honor, and folly into wisdom. According to its doctrine, this can be achieved by cultivating the Buddha nature within each individual.

You may ask if it is even necessary to adopt this goal if, by comparison, your life situation is negligible in relation to the immense suffering of many around the world. How can you compare your frustrations, for example, to the lack of food and daily comfort of others?

Buddhism is truly democratic in response. The belief that all life is connected and interrelated is the abiding premise that answers the question. While the relativity of suffering is understood, its nature is universal and its causes return to the three poisons. One person's emotional anguish is as much a cause of suffering as another's lack of shelter.

How does meditation address suffering? Buddhists say that by cultivating the Buddha nature, an individual develops the insights to discover the causes of suffering in his own life. Then, the student can come to terms with those causes and learn the means to eliminate them. It cannot be found in dogmas or methods but requires the individual to begin the journey to these discoveries, using Buddhist principles only as guideposts.

FACT

The *sutra* ("thread, string") is a scripture containing one of the teachings of the Buddha. Some of the *sutras* are regarded as more important than others, such as the *Heart Sutra*, the *Sutra of Innumerable Meanings*, and the *Lotus Sutra*.

Buddhism and the West

Many who studied Buddhism in depth when it was introduced to the West in the mid-twentieth century saw its value to contemporary society. The adaptation of Buddhist philosophy to Western life, they believed, introduced a new form of psychology. The goals are the same—integration and wholeness—and its purpose is to help you observe how you treat yourself. That viewpoint was quite accurate, because Buddhism has attracted a large number of psychology professionals—analysts, therapists, and psychologists. They agree that Buddhism offers some fundamental approaches to self-awareness and the development of healthy attitudes.

Buddhist Meditation

A central teaching of Buddhism is that enlightenment is attained through persistent practice. And the practice that embodies this teaching is *dhyana* ("meditation"). The goal can be reached by emulating the Buddha when he reached enlightenment—sitting in meditation.

There is no single approach in Buddhist meditation, however. There are many approaches, and each school offers a variation on meditation practice. One characteristic of all schools is the emphasis on mindfulness. This state is the complete awareness of the immediate in time and the reality presented by the senses. It means apprehending body, feelings, mind, and the environment in unison. We may assume that this is the way we are all the time, even now. But Buddhism points out that most of what we assume to be reality is an illusion, brought about by the wrong use of body, feelings, mind, and the environment.

Another characteristic of Buddhist meditation is the emphasis on overcoming attachments. That's because the problems that arise from this are manifold, in the individual and in society. Now, this does not mean denying "attachment" to a loved one, a faithful pet, or a reliable automobile. In fact, Buddhism encourages feelings of devotion, compassion, and appreciation. But there are some things in every life that really don't bring out our true nature. For example, a relationship that is based not on love but on mutual dependency is an attachment. A pet that you have no time for is an attachment. And an expensive automobile that stays in your garage is an attachment.

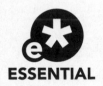

ESSENTIAL

Control of mental processes is also a characteristic of Buddhist meditation. One technique is analytical meditation. Here, the meditator counters fleeting thoughts or images with affirmations of the goal that he wishes to attain (and it should ultimately be enlightenment). This is a process of continually training the mind to stay with a focal point each time it begins to stray.

Meditation to overcome attachments can resolve these problems. Here, a three-pronged approach is used:

1. **Anatman:** Viewing all attachments as abstractions that do not exist in their own right. Instead, they are part of the realm of *maya* (illusion) that is neither undesirable nor attractive (neither negative nor positive).
2. **Anitya:** Contemplating the impermanence of all attachments in life. In other words, these things will come and go; they will change, break down, or go their own way eventually. They are subject to the endless cycle as is everything else.

3. **Duhkha:** Realizing that attachments are the cause of suffering. This realization even includes attachments that bring pleasure; they will cause suffering because they will eventually end.

Since Buddhist meditation emphasizes mindfulness to a large extent, you may want to develop the ability to achieve this state. You can do this anywhere the opportunity or desire presents itself. You are not going to formally meditate, but you'll exercise some of your meditative senses, which could lead to entering the meditative state.

Choose one of your external senses: hearing, seeing, tasting, touching, or smelling. Whatever presents itself to you, use that sense to completely "rediscover" what presents itself at the moment.

Allow an ordinary daily event to use your external sense. Let this little event be the only focus of your attention, for as long as it lasts. For example, you may be standing over the stove, stirring soup for lunch. Using one of your senses you might:

- Listen for the sounds of steam, bubbling liquid, and stirring.
- Observe the motion of the liquid as it heats and is stirred, watching the ingredients change texture and color.
- Taste the soup slowly and periodically, noticing changes in flavor and temperature.
- Distinguish the variations in scent as the soup is heated, cooled, and tasted.

Buddhist Contradictions

It is not uncommon to discover contradictions in some Buddhist ideas, but these are often used as springboards for meditation. For example, the idea of *maya*, or illusion, expresses the deceptive nature of external life and the world of the senses. The outer reality is not immutable, according to this view, and has no relation to the "ultimate reality." At the same time, one may enter into a meditative state where the external senses are closely observed in their interaction with the external world. If the world is an illusion, you might ask, what is the point of using the senses to monitor that illusion?

This is one of those "Aha!" moments that some branches of Buddhism seek, such as traditional Zen and modern insight approaches. Some things seem irreconcilable and nonsensical in both the outer and the inner worlds. With the practice of meditation, however, impossible contradictions can make sense. The goal here is to transcend the dualities of what is real and what is not real, and reach true reality. What could that be? For those who are alleged to have reached it, it is a world of pure love. For others, it is pure laughter. In other words, it is pure contradiction.

Buddhist Luminaries

Allan Bennett (1872–1923) was one of the first English scholars to travel to the East and study Buddhism and bring its teachings back to the West. He lived in Sri Lanka (Ceylon) and Burma, and wrote several books, including *Outline of Buddhism*. He was strongly influenced in this direction by the journalist-poet Sir Edwin Arnold (1832–1904), author of *The Light of Asia*.

FACT

Jack Kornfield is cofounder of the Insight Meditation Society in Barre, Massachusetts. He studied Buddhism in India and taught different styles of meditation at the California Esalen Institute and Denver's Naropa Institute in the 1970s. His widely read book, *A Still Forest Pool*, is a rich source of meditation guidance in the vipassana tradition.

Thich Nhat Hanh is a Vietnamese monk who was nominated for the Nobel Peace Prize by Martin Luther King Jr. A student at New York's Columbia University, he returned to Vietnam at the close of the war to assist in projects of reconciliation and social service. Although his approach falls within the Zen style of Buddhism, he has written much on the value of peaceful social action and coined the term *engaged Buddhism*. It is an approach to putting Buddhist practice into everyday, meaningful work for society.

CHAPTER 10

The Road to Shambhala: Tibetan Buddhism

The mighty Himalayan peaks birthed a rich Buddhist tradition with its own forms of music, dance, ritual, and art, an entire culture designed to support meditation. Although the Chinese government has sought to undermine these practices, the political repression in Tibet has paradoxically helped to spread knowledge of Tibetan Buddhism throughout the world. In this chapter, you will gain wisdom from this vital tradition to support your meditation practice.

The Tibetan Buddhist Tradition

Each of us has a mystical instinct that is expressed in subtle, everyday events. Lighting a candle always elicits a reverent hush, while the scent of incense warms the senses. In a similar way, the resonating ring of a bell brings clarity of thought, while the image of a deity evokes fascination and respect.

We need this mystical dimension, or we would lose our sense of wonder. It offers enrichment to mind and body, making the efforts we spend in thought and action meaningful. Mystical meditation is a way of approaching this dimension confidently, allowing us to experience the inner life in profound ways.

FACT

Although he was not the first to do so, the Dalai Lama broke from the isolation that had culturally sequestered Tibet from the rest of Asia. He initiated a continuing dialogue with other religious leaders, followers, and governments after his exile. In time, Tibetan monasteries opened in England, Scotland, France, and the United States, to provide continuity to a culture without borders.

Interest in the culture and religion of Tibet became widespread in the mid-twentieth century, mostly due to the forced exile of the country's spiritual leader, the fourteenth Dalai Lama. The fate of this young monk, who is also regarded as the secular head of the country, was recounted by a number of travelers who managed to enter the forbidden zones of the Himalayas and the closely guarded capital of Lhasa in the 1940s and 1950s. At the time, the Chinese occupied the region, suppressing Tibetan culture and religion. The core of Tibet's spiritual practice is a unique branch of Mahayana Buddhism, strongly blended with the indigenous folk religion, Bon-po.

Buddhism Comes to Tibet

Mahayana Buddhism came to Tibet between the seventh and eighth centuries. For a thousand years, it had been spreading from India northward to China, Korea, and Japan, but it failed to take hold in Tibet early because of the country's isolation and strong entrenchment in Bon-po, the native religion. This is one of the more fascinating aspects of Tibetan culture and is responsible for making its Buddhist heritage so unique. This combination of a great tradition with indigenous beliefs has created an approach to meditation that is fascinating and attractive to many Westerners.

Tibetan Magic and Medicine

Astrology, divination, and alchemy are also integrated into Tibetan Buddhist practice. They are viewed as skillful means, a term used by the Buddha to encourage the use of all approaches that assist in attaining enlightenment. They, in turn, influenced a centuries-old tradition of medical practice that has caught the attention of Western healers. Tibetan medicine combines a skilled knowledge of surgery and of pharmacology derived from herbal medicine. Tibetan healers maintain another interesting approach to understanding the psychic origins of disease. They carefully observe dreams and omens to provide clues to both the causes and cures of most illnesses. The healers seek an understanding of all dimensions of the person's life and use those skills that meditation promotes. Observation, attention, mindfulness, and compassion are the cornerstones to good health and longevity.

Demons, Deities, and Ghosts

The father or Guru Rinpoche ("great guru") of Tibetan Buddhism is known as Padmasambhava, "born of the lotus." Living in the northwest region of India in the eighth century in what is now Pakistan, he was an esteemed Tantric *siddha,* or master of Yogic practice. Legend says that he was called to Tibet by the monarch Thi-Srong to exorcise the region of interfering demons, believed to be opposing the spread of Buddhism in Tibet. The holy man used his masterful skills to tame those demons, and they became the "dharma protectors" of Tibet's religion. For example, Tara is one of the indigenous goddess figures, a form of the divine mother. Also viewed as a protector, she merged into the Buddhist stream that entered Tibet. To this day, Tara is honored through images, special ceremonies, and festivals.

Tibetan art and iconography depicts these figures in great detail and with much power. They attest to the fusion of folk magic with Buddhist philosophy.

Since the migration of the Tibetan people from their native country to India, a wealth of art has been exported to appreciative collectors and museums throughout the world. Fifty years ago, Tibetan art was extremely rare; today it can be seen in every major museum in the West. Affordable folk art of the same caliber can be acquired just about anywhere.

But why is the sublime philosophy of Buddhism expressed in such powerful and sometimes frightening ways? Elaborate pictures of wrathful deities, hungry ghosts, and guardian demons are alien to the Western mind. They seem to contradict the message of serenity and celestial harmony that the Tibetan doctrine means to espouse. So, what's wrong with this picture?

Bon-po is a Tibetan expression of shamanism, the belief in communicating with the forces in nature and in divine realms. A pantheon of gods and goddesses represents these forces, which may be assumed by the shaman or practitioner. Certain rituals, prayers, and practices (such as wearing amulets) are believed to strengthen the bond between the believer and the divine force.

The Tibetan Buddhist sees these images as metaphors. Benevolent and wrathful images speak of impersonal forces in the living universe, but they also represent human qualities that must be met and defused. In meditation, we may encounter feelings of jealousy, anger, and frustration. By externalizing these emotions we are better able to detach from them, but this is not necessarily a process of expressing them. Instead, it can be a process of visualization and inner dialogue with the image. In other words, we don't have to throw knives at a target in order to feel revenge. Instead, we can meditate on the image of revenge and become acquainted with it fully, understand it, and make peace with it.

Branches of Tibetan Buddhism

Padmasambhava's teachings formed the foundation of Tibet's monastic movement. At the time the Chinese invasion of the country began in 1957, members of the monastic communities comprised nearly half the population. The Tibetans regard their approach to Buddhism as Vajrayana, the "diamond vehicle." It accommodates both the magical theme of Bon-po with the philosophical theme of Buddhism. What distinguishes Vajrayana Buddhism from other schools is an emphasis on initiations and empowerments, performed by meditation masters. Such masters are experienced in mystical and reserved forms of meditation that require special instructions and a lot of practice.

Over the centuries, aspects of Buddhist teaching particular to Tibet branched off and established separate practices. Three schools of teachings, still prevalent today, were established by the eleventh century. They have their own monasteries, courses of study, and monastic rules of behavior. They are not adversarial either in precept or spirit, but they do emphasize differing perspectives that are believed by each school to be most important in spiritual growth.

Nyingmapa ("Old Ones")

This branch is also known as the Red Hats, from the ceremonial headdresses worn by their lamas. They teach a mystically oriented practice, with much emphasis on Tantric ritual. Nine *yamas* ("limbs") to enlightenment make up the teachings of this school. The oldest monastic order in Tibet, Nyingmapa's lineage is traced to Guru Rinpoche. This branch emphasizes solitary meditation with a type of practice known as *dzogchen*, the "great perfection" meditation. Its goal is attainment of the primordial state of being, which forms the core of all conscious activity. The Red Hats eat meat and do not reject sexuality, which they see as another means to enlightenment.

Kagyupa ("Transmitters of the Word")

This branch is also known as the Black Hats. Following the Guru Rinpoche, the Indian Buddhist teacher Naropa trained a number of disciples in India, who traveled to Tibet and established this lineage. The most regarded text on the Kagyu meditation system is the *Mahamudra*, written in the sixteenth century by Wang Ch'ug Dorje. It outlines the teaching of mindfulness meditation, training the mind to be focused on the moment with all conscious faculties.

Gelugpa ("Virtuous Ones")

This branch is also known as the Yellow Hats. This school emphasizes philosophical study and ascetic practices, including a meditation practice that is mastered in graduated stages. The Dalai Lamas are heads of this school, and since the seventeenth century have ruled the country of Tibet from its capital at Lhasa. The current Dalai Lama is viewed as the fourteenth incarnation of Gendun-drup, a fourteenth-century disciple of Tsong Kha-pa, who founded the lineage. The Yellow Hats reject sexuality as a means to enlightenment and introduced vegetarianism in Tibetan life.

Sakyapa ("Gray Earth Ones")

This branch is named for their monastic center in southern Tibet. An intellectual tradition, the Sakyapa has archived Tantric writings since its inception in the eleventh century. The head of this school is the Sakya Tri-zin, who inherits the title from his uncle and is always a member of the Khon family line. The lineage traces its connection back to the thirteenth century, to the great Mongol emperor of China, the Kublai Khan.

FACT

Although study of sacred texts and the learning of ancient prayers to the Buddhas and bodhisattvas encompass much of monastic training, the practitioner is not required to commit to extended study. Thus, like all other Buddhist practices, meditation forms the core of action that leads to fulfilling both the spiritual and practical goals of the student.

Modern Tibetan Buddhism

Because the Tibetan tradition has fused the cultural richness of the region with Buddhist philosophy, its meditation style reflects this unique synthesis. What you may see in a Tibetan Buddhist practice will differ from the Zen Buddhist practice, even though the goals are essentially the same:

- To awaken the Buddha nature within the individual
- To develop compassion for the suffering in the world
- To discover a means of alleviating the suffering that is perceived

In keeping with its classical Buddhist roots, Tibetan Buddhism is focused on the dharma ("law, teachings of the Buddha"), specifically on meditation as the means of alleviating suffering.

Good Karma, Bad Karma

Karma is the Sanskrit word for "action," no more, no less. The Buddhist doctrine of karma holds that every intentional act (physical, verbal, and mental) leaves an imprint or residue. Like a seed, that residue will proliferate, eventually having an effect at some future point. That effect will be infused with pleasure or pain for the person, depending on the nature of the past act. Ten nonvirtuous deeds will determine this:

- Covetousness
- Divisive speech
- Harmful intent
- Harsh speech
- Killing
- Lying
- Senseless speech
- Sexual misconduct
- Stealing
- Wrong view

In Buddhism, there is truly no "good" or "bad" karma, merely the result of a previous action. That is why meditation is so important. Through it, the qualities of mindfulness and compassion are developed. When that takes place, nonvirtuous deeds become rare, if not impossible. The resulting karma will be virtuous.

Tibetan Buddhist Luminaries

In modern times, a number of influential Tibetan Buddhist teachers came to America to "spread the dharma," or disseminate the teachings of the Buddha.

Chogyam Trungpa (1939–1987), of the Kagyupa lineage, came to study in Great Britain in the 1960s. He made a deep, permanent impact on spiritual practice in the West. He initially helped establish the first Tibetan Buddhist center in Scotland and subsequently founded the Naropa Institute in Boulder, Colorado. A prolific writer, Trungpa wrote of the "spiritual materialism" that pervaded the times, and how the practice of meditation could be a remedy to the thousand ills of modern life.

The Dalai Lama is of the Gelugpa lineage. Born Tenzin Gyatso in 1935, he is regarded as a living bodhisattva, the manifestation of Chenrezi, "the compassionate one." But he is also a teacher and leader of the Tibetan people, both religiously and politically. Forced into exile in 1959, he received the Nobel Peace Prize in 1989 for his nonviolent opposition to the Chinese occupation of Tibet. In addition to his political efforts, he lectures and writes prolifically on meditation and the practice of active compassion in everyday life.

A brave pilgrim and world traveler, Alexandra David-Neel (1868–1969) was the first Western woman to enter Tibet in the twentieth century. Born in France, she embarked on meetings with scholars and philosophers in the Orient at a time when their existence was barely known in the West. She learned the Tibetan language, studied in several monasteries, and adopted a lama as a son. Throughout her long life, most of her work was devoted to producing books that opened the portal to Tibetan culture and wisdom.

Creating a Tibetan Buddhist Shrine

Most Buddhist practices incorporate a shrine that becomes the meeting point between the individual meditator and the object of meditation. Here, the object is the Buddha, but this is not a prayer- or worship-oriented practice. Rather, the Buddha is a universal image that is used as a focus, the embodiment of the goal. Different images of the Buddha represent different qualities of the mind that were attained by the Buddha and that can be cultivated by the meditator.

The Reason Behind the Shrine

In the Tibetan approach, the creation and care of the shrine is a meditation in itself. This is another expression of the Tantric theme, the "ritual path" to enlightenment. Setting up a shrine follows certain guidelines, which you may adapt to your own space and daily agenda. Once you have established the routine, it is difficult to abandon. There is something timeless about cleaning and caring for a sacred space, especially when it is one of your own making. This is part of the beauty of Tibetan meditation practice, and it teaches the value of simple, mindful activity.

FACT

In the Tantric path, which Tibetan meditation espouses, the shrine is a symbol, a tangible means of expressing the goal of meditation. It is a reminder, a source of inspiration, and a focus for your meditation activity. Most important, the shrine is a space dedicated to your own spirit, your higher self—what you are striving to become.

Where to Put the Shrine

The shrine should be in a place that is above the waist, or higher than the seat that will be used in meditation. Place the image or picture of the Buddha in the highest spot, and all other objects will be placed below it or off to the side. Seven offering bowls are traditional to the Tibetan shrine. Candles and flowers may surround the image, and offerings of food (fruit and grain are best), incense, and water are traditionally offered. In some households, the first plate of food in a daily meal is offered, and then returned to the kitchen for distribution.

The Sitting Space

Meditation in this practice is performed sitting on the floor before the shrine. Colorful wool Tibetan carpets, woven with the traditional images of dragon, lion, and tiger, can be placed on the floor. They serve as a reminder of the animal powers that are both evoked and mastered in the meditation process. Over that, support cushions may be placed, either the *zabuton* (mat) and *zafu* (round pillow), or a *gomden*. The latter is a firm, rectangular cushion that provides extra lift and support for beginners and is favored in Tibetan meditation practice.

Most Tibetan meditation sessions begin with the reading of sacred texts. As a preliminary exercise, this prepares the mind by freeing it from mundane thoughts and focusing on the meditation itself. For this, the *chog-tse* ("practice table") is placed on the floor before the meditator to support the various sheets of printed texts. Prayer beads and cups of tea, which are allowed through meditation, may also rest on the practice table. The traditional dimensions of the table, made of three simple finished pieces of wood, are 11 inches wide, 28 inches in length, and 13 inches high.

Accessories to Include in the Shrine

The Tibetan meditation shrine embodies the two approaches unique to this tradition: meditation and ritual. Elaborate shrines may also include other symbolic accessories. The bell and *dorje* are two ritual implements representing the feminine principle of wisdom (bell) and the masculine principle of compassionate action (*dorje*, or *vajra*). The *dorje* is a scepter or wand that represents a fiery thunderbolt. They are offered at the shrine before meditation as sound and music, respectively.

Kata is the white scarf that is presented and received as an offering. Made of gauze-like cotton, it symbolizes purity of intention. Offerings that are made to gurus are given with the *kata* or it may be presented alone. A *kata* received from a revered teacher may be worn by the student at gatherings or in meditation.

Mala is the Tibetan rosary or beaded necklace used in meditation. It usually contains 27 beads (for prostrations) and 108 beads (for mantra). Different precious stones used for the *mala* beads are associated with various aspects of the Buddha or bodhisattvas. For instance, lapis lazuli is associated with the Medicine ("healing") Buddha, and pink coral with the Amitabha ("universal love") Buddha. Used for counting, the *mala* is held in the left hand between the thumb and forefinger. It may be worn around the neck or kept in a special bag when not in use.

The prayer wheel is a circular compartment on a rod that turns clockwise as it is spun. Within the wheel are wound written mantras that send blessings in the "ten directions," to all sentient beings as they spin. Fabricated of wood, bamboo, copper, and silver, many Buddhist prayer wheels are works of art and may range in size from a child's toy to the enormous stationary wheels in Nepal that require several persons to turn.

The *stupa* is a tiered structure usually with a lotiform crown that in miniature form serves as a reliquary for sacred objects. It represents the mind of the Buddha, with its many ascending layers of awakening and enlightenment. Throughout India, ancient *stupas* are found in sacred places where the Buddha's relics are believed buried. In the Orient, *stupas* are known as pagodas.

The *thangka* is a colorful embroidered image of the Buddha, idealized gurus, or bodhisattvas. Usually made of silk, they are hung on the walls surrounding the shrine. These images represent enlightened qualities and help engage the imagination, an important component in this school of meditation.

Caring for the Shrine

The floor of the shrine room should always be swept clean, and it is customary to go barefoot in the space. While sitting in meditation, point the feet away from the shrine.

It is customary to "open" the shrine in the morning and "close" it in the evening. When opening, fresh offerings are provided, and when closing, they are removed and the accessories are cleaned. These little events provide openings for meditation, even if they are brief.

Meditation on the Supreme Mantra

Unique to this tradition are two revered devices: the image of Chenrezi, the Tibetan form of Avalokitesvara (also known as "regarder of the cries of the world") and his mantra, *Om-mani-padme-hum*. Chenrezi means "looking with clear eyes," and he represents the prototype of compassion that the meditator aspires to.

The recitation of the mantra not only evokes this bodhisattva, it is viewed as a means to reaching the mind of enlightenment. *Om-mani-padme-hum* is commonly interpreted as "Behold the jewel in the lotus." Whole books have been written on its mystic meaning. It is essentially a synonym for the fusion of the active and passive divine principles (*lingam-yoni* or masculine-feminine). This is once more an allusion to the sexual imagery in Tantric Buddhism that expresses a universe in a continual state of creation.

A World of Peace

A Buddhist text of great importance in the Tibetan tradition is the *Kalachakra Tantra*. In it, an allegorical tale is disclosed:

In the kingdom of Shambhala, far north of the Himalayas, the Buddha entrusted a valuable tantra (teaching) to its king, the Kalkin. The region is shaped like a giant lotus, filled with sandalwood forests and lotus lakes, and it is encircled by snowy peaks. Kalapa, the capital, features a powerful mandala in the middle of the city, the Buddha Kalachakra. Here, there is freedom from sickness and poverty, and all who live there are intelligent and virtuous. Those who are reborn there attain Buddhahood.

But in the year 2425, demons and barbarians will set out to invade Shambhala. Then, the 25th Kalkin, Raudracakrin, will lead his armies out of the kingdom to meet the forces of evil in an apocalyptic battle, from which Buddhism will emerge victorious. This will usher in an age when the human lifespan will increase, crops will grow without being cultivated, and the earth will devote itself to the practice of Buddhism.

Adapted from *Prisoners of Shangri-La* by Donald S. Lopez, Jr. (University of Chicago Press; 1998)

This mythical story is believed to be the prophecy of an actual event, one that is unfolding in our present age. To protect those who are meant to reside in Shambhala, the protection and benefit of the Buddha Kalachakra is transmitted through a sublime empowerment, the Kalachakra initiation. It has only become accessible in modern times, since the beginning of the Tibetan diaspora to the West in the middle of the twentieth century. This empowerment is believed to pacify all conflicts and promote peace, for both the practitioner and the community where it is performed.

Peace Meditation

One of the meditation prayers recited in the Kalachakra empowerment asks the Buddha of compassion for these benefits:

May there be no untimely death, illness,
Or obstructing spirits for us.
May we have no nightmares,
Ill omens, or bad dealings.
May the world enjoy peace, have good harvests,
Abundant grain, the growth of dharma.
May we have glorious auspiciousness,
To accomplish whatever mind desires.

Attending a Kalachakra empowerment is a rare occasion. If the opportunity presents itself, do not miss it. The empowerment takes place over a period of five days, and is truly a "meditation celebration." In between teachings given by Tibetan lamas, meditation sessions are held and ceremonies honor the bodhisattvas that bring peace and enlightenment.

QUOTE

"As you progress in your meditation, you get to a point where you loosen your grip. Your attitude becomes more flexible and you realize the absence of an intrinsic independent reality of phenomena."
—The Dalai Lama

Meditation on Emptiness

The ultimate goal in Tibetan meditation is attainment of the *mahamudra* ("great seal"), known as the "realization of emptiness." Here, the meditator enters the Buddha mind, approaching through *shi-nay* ("meditation on emptiness"). In it, the meditator undergoes a process of becoming empty of independent identity, in order to realize the primordial state of being. What does this mean and how is it done?

Identity is a phenomenon of mind, and this is the object of meditation. Emptiness in this context does not mean that everything we possess in the mind is not "real" or has no meaning. Rather, it means that the true nature of mind is transparent, a reflection of something else. And that something else can only be known by taking the journey to reach it through meditation.

The *mahamudra* is a practice closely associated with the Kagyupa lineage. It is a lifelong quest and the subject of profound teachings in Tibetan Buddhism. The preparatory practices that lead to its discovery take time and much meditation experience.

The Tibetan Book of the Dead

How could a "book of the dead" be associated with meditation? Most ancient cultures have sacred texts concerning the passage of life into invisible realms. They are found in Egypt, India, Africa, and the Americas. Their purpose is to guide a person through those invisible realms, to be at peace, and to meet with the deity.

The *Bardo Thodol* is Tibet's book of the dead, a sacred text in the keeping of the Nyingmapa lineage. Bardo means "the in-between state" or transition. In this philosophy, there are six *bardos;* the first three exist in our conscious world: birth, dreaming, and meditation. The second set of bardos represents the states entered after death. They are the moment of death, the supreme reality, and the state of becoming.

Thodol means "liberation through hearing." As the name suggests, the text is intended to liberate the soul from its earthly ties to enter the white light of supreme reality. For a period of forty-nine days, passages of the book are recited on behalf of the soul, so it may be guided through the in-between states.

However, the *Bardo Thodol* is an important meditation guide. It outlines a map for entering higher states, for those who wish to go "beyond death." It has been used in modern times as a psychoanalytic tool and a healing text.

A Tibetan Tea Break

Conditions in the high, cold atmosphere of the Himalayas led to the custom of drinking buttered tea. The Tibetans regard it as a life-extending drink and internal cleanser. It is still regarded by meditators as an excellent way to sharpen the mind while relaxing the body.

The key ingredient, butter, should be clarified. To clarify the butter, gently warm it to melting (you can use a microwave or a heated skillet). The clear, yellow liquid butter is then separated from the white butterfat globules that come to rest at the bottom. The clear liquid is what is used in making the tea. In most Eastern import grocery stores, jars of clarified butter, known as *ghee,* are sold at reasonable cost. It is the most common cooking oil used in Indian and Pakistani dishes. Here's a recipe for two cups; you may use decaffeinated tea if you prefer.

Buttered Tea

1 teaspoon of strong black tea leaves or 1 tea bag (Ceylon, Darjeeling, or gunpowder)

1½ cups very cold water

½ cup milk (regular or low fat)

1 teaspoon clarified butter

Add the tea to the water in a small pan and bring it to a boil, simmer for a few minutes, then add the milk. Heat to nearly, but not quite, boiling, then remove from the stove and add the clarified butter. Whisk for about a minute, then strain it into a cup.

CHAPTER 11

Energy and Balance

You may want to know how it's possible to balance the activities that fill each day. Allotting time to work, play, and rest is one way, but being tied to a schedule is not conducive to true relaxation. Discovering the source of energy is the real challenge, and some meditation traditions answer that in interesting ways.

The Way of the Tao

Many of us seek meditation to restore our energy levels. The demands of daily living scatter our energies, from the mental concentration required by our jobs to the physical tasks of errands and housekeeping. Physical fitness is another necessity that many of us pursue to remedy the one-sidedness of life, but that often diminishes the feeling of vitality, too. Some fitness programs foster an atmosphere of competition, so that "keeping up" is the only way you think you can succeed. Small wonder that low energy is a common complaint of modern life.

Taoist philosophy relates to just this situation. It predates both Confucianism ("tradition of scholars") and Buddhism. Originating in ancient China, Taoism espouses mystical meditation and other practices that encourage the discovery and development of inner power.

FACT

Tao simply means "the way." It alludes to both the path that is followed for physical, mental, and spiritual balance, and the energy it is composed of. It is a continuous, living process.

Some believe that the origin of Taoism lies in the shamanic heritage of ancient China, just as Bon-po represents the shamanic expression of Tibet. There is certainly much evidence to support this. All of the components of Taoism have a mystical basis, a belief in the living, conscious aspect of all life. It is eternal and universal, and returning to it brings the practitioner to the source of vitality. The essential practice, then, is to join with or "become one" with the Tao.

Cosmology and the Human Body

Like all the great traditions, Taoism views the life force as a continuously moving, vitalizing energy. It penetrates everywhere and everything. This force, *ch'i* ("breath" or "energy"), is the basis for a comprehensive philosophy. It is the key principle in Asian medicine, martial arts, spiritual practice, art, and architecture.

Ch'i is subject to two currents that are in continuous interplay in the universe: yin and yang. These currents create the visible world and affect everything, from the genesis of galaxies to the renewal of cells in the human body. A knowledge of how, when, and where the yin and yang forces work is the essence of Taoist philosophy and meditation. With this knowledge, the practitioner can maintain serenity of mind, health of body, and harmony with nature.

▼ YIN AND YANG ASSOCIATIONS

Realm	Yang	Yin
Cosmic	Heaven	Earth
Luminary	Sun	Moon
Seasons	Summer, spring	Winter, autumn
Temperature	Dry	Damp
Gender	Masculine	Feminine
Colors	Red	Black
Animal	Dragon	Tiger
Visual	Light	Dark
Time	Day	Night
Taste	Salt	Sweet

Yin and yang are in continual flux. If they were to stop, the visible universe would no longer exist, except for *ch'i*, which would be in a state of suspension.

In the body, *ch'i* flows through a network of natural pathways called meridians. The consistent passage of *ch'i* through these meridians is necessary for harmonious living on all levels. Sophisticated techniques have been devised to remedy any blockages or stagnation that may occur. You may be familiar with some of these techniques. The individual may undertake the practice of *t'ai chi* ("supreme energy") and *t'ai chi ch'uan* ("supreme fist method"), combining meditative practice with beneficial physical movement. Acupuncture, moxibustion, massage, or herbal treatment are healing techniques used to restore the function of the meridians.

In nature, *ch'i* is also of great consequence. In places where it is blocked or stagnant, there will be no proliferation of life. As a result, animals and people may become ill and crops will not grow. To make matters worse, undesirable ghosts and nature spirits may congregate, creating more bad *ch'i. Feng shui* ("wind and water") is a practice or treatment that aims at harmonizing the environment.

The Pa Kua

The movement and balance of yin and yang is expressed in the *Pa Kua* cosmic diagram. This image depicts the life force in all eight possible manifestations. In the depiction, Yang is a straight line, representing the direct force. Yin is a broken line, representing the yielding force. Yang and yin are inseparable: When one overtakes, the other will seek balance by overtaking. Thus, each has three innate conditions: direct, yielding, and balance. These three conditions comprise the trigrams. There are eight possible trigrams, each one a combination of yang and yin in the three conditions. They are arranged around a center (the universe) depicting their various manifestations.

The *Pa Kua* is an excellent tool for use in meditation. Its eight sides represent the balance of the yang-yin forces through the motion of the trigrams.

Individually, the eight trigrams represent meditative states. They may be inscribed on paper or written on cards to use in meditation sessions. Each trigram is a key to balance of mind through images that represent universal conditions. The trigrams are:

1. *Ch'ien* ("the creative") is the heavenly father, spirit. Here there is strength, resolve, and motion forward.
2. *Li* ("the depending") is the clinging fire, radiance. Become aroused to dedication, perseverance, and dependence on the inspirational.
3. *Tui* ("the joyous lake") is the water that nourishes everyone. Here there is cause for joy and relinquishing hardship; what has been given is returned.
4. *Sun* ("the gentle") is returning to a familiar place. Influence the outer reality and gain control of it through gentleness.
5. *K'un* ("the receptive") is the earthly mother, nature. This is the experience of devotion, gentleness, and duration.
6. *K'an* ("the grotto") is entering a hidden place. When danger presents itself, withdraw and find respite in natural surroundings.

7. *Kên* ("the mountain") is keeping still. When attaining goals, pause to prepare for the next advance.
8. *Chên* ("the arousing") is movement and thunder. By putting the self in order, excitement builds and laughter breaks the tension.

The I Ching

The combination of the eight trigrams in pairs gives rise to the sixty-four hexagrams of the *I Ching* ("*Book of Changes*"). It is a book of wisdom and an oracular tool that allegedly dates from 2800 B.C.E. This is the time of its legendary author Fu Hsi, the first of China's noble emperors. In some Taoist temples, he is shown holding the eight trigrams, which he is believed to have invented.

The *I Ching* is an important source of ancient Chinese philosophy in the Taoist tradition. In it, the sixty-four hexagrams present all of the possible conditions and experiences that individuals may face at critical periods. The text provides insights into these events and the means by which they can be altered; hence, the "changes." Besides consulting the *I Ching* when counsel is needed, a practitioner may seek guidance as part of a daily meditation. A mindful approach is called for in order to acquire a clear picture of the present circumstances and future possibilities.

Taoist Luminaries

Important historical figures are revered in Taoism. Among them is its greatest philosopher, Lao Tzu, who wrote the *Tao-te Ching* ("*The Book of the Way and Its Power*"). From this work, which consists of 5,000 pictograms assembled in the second century B.C.E., the basis of Taoist philosophy and religion is presented.

Lao Tzu promoted the practice of *ch'i kung* ("working with energy"). It is a meditative system of breathing that progressively leads to "the return to the Tao." From this practice came many of the meditative and martial arts disciplines of China, including *kung fu,* taught at the legendary Shao-lin monastery. In modern times it has been presented to the West in its healing form under the name of *qigong* ("chi kung").

The Discovery of Ch'i in the West

In the early twentieth century, the German-born neuropsychiatrist Wilhelm Reich proposed that life energy not only exists, it can be harnessed. He called his discovery orgone energy, and he spent many years analyzing and experimenting with it. One of his inventions was the orgone box, which looked like a sitting sauna enclosure. It was meant to accumulate, balance, and pass the orgone into the sitter. Reich's fellow scientists dismissed the work, however. He was persecuted in the press and died tragically in 1957. Subsequently, his work was revived and used as a basis for the development of bioenergetics and Rolfing, Western approaches to releasing blocked energy in the human body and restoring psychological well-being.

QUOTE

"One yin, one yang, that is the Tao."

—*The Book of Changes*

In another discipline, physicist Fritjof Capra, author of *The Tao of Physics,* draws together the empirical world of scientific research and traditional meditation. The nature of reality, he says, is expressed as much in Taoist philosophy as in the most recent models of the universe.

Inner Alchemy

In Taoism, the human body is seen as a microcosm of the universe. Within it flows *ch'i,* pulsating to the rhythms of the yin and yang currents. Naturally, an individual's balance and harmony will dictate how this flow will affect her, physically and mentally. Techniques for ensuring balance and harmony are taught for meditation, healing, and physical and mental development.

Nei Tan is a branch of Taoism that is concerned with the transformation of the body and the development of the soul. Its principal approach is alchemy, but this is not the legendary practice of the Middle Ages that attempted to turn lead into gold. Rather, it is a spiritual practice, using the symbolic language of alchemy to represent inner, mystical processes.

In this system, three vital centers of the body are visualized as the "three cinnabar fields." Cinnabar is a highly valued reddish mineral (mercuric sulfide) in China. You may have seen sculpture from Asia fabricated from cinnabar, usually carved elaborately with figures of dragons and phoenixes.

ESSENTIAL

The practice of Nei Tan is twofold: the *ch'i* is purified within the body, while all mechanisms of thought are brought under perfect control. The goal is achieved through meditative exercises that harmonize the three vital energies possessed by human beings. These are *ch'i* ("energy"), *ching* ("essence"), and *shen* ("spirit"). Another way to look at these vital energies is that they represent mind, body, and the immortal soul.

The cinnabar fields represent the centers where the combined movements of yin and yang take place in the body. Within the cinnabar fields, thousands of deities reside. They govern the organs and preserve their functions so the life force may remain in the body.

The lower cinnabar field is at the navel, the *tan t'ien*. Here are the forces that govern reproduction and the prolongation of life. The middle cinnabar field is in the chest, the *ch'i hai* ("ocean of breath"). The upper cinnabar field is in the brain, *ni huan* ("ball of clay"). It is the residence of the highest deity of the body and the ultimate recipient of *ch'i* in its most refined form.

Taoist Healing

In Taoist philosophy, most disease is viewed as arising from erroneous living. There are seven emotional factors cited as the causes of disease: anger, fear, fright, grief, joy, sorrow, and worry.

Meditation can prevent these factors from draining the body of *ch'i*. The meditator can detach from powerful emotions that accumulate in the body and cause illness.

Another consideration is the quality of *ch'i* in the environment. Taoists believe that living *ch'i* is present from midnight to noon, the yang period of the day. Conversely, dead *ch'i* is in circulation from noon to midnight, the yin period of the day. Thus, breathing exercises are taken in the most vital half of the day.

Unblocking Energy

One way to begin on this transformative path is to practice *Tao Yin* ("stretching and contracting"). It is identical in spirit to Hatha Yoga and is very simple to accomplish. Its purpose is to unblock the *ch'i* in the body before beginning deep meditation.

Observation of the body's actions and reactions must be directed in each of the eight steps that are performed repetitively for one minute each while standing:

1. **Clapping:** This applies to all motions the body can make in bringing together the pairs—clapping hands, clicking the teeth together, raising and lowering the heels to tap the floor. Maintain a gentle rhythm.
2. **Turning:** Turn your shoulders to the left while turning the head to the right; then reverse the action. Move slowly and deliberately.
3. **Stirring:** Rotate your tongue around your mouth cavity, taking care to keep the mouth closed; then allow it to touch the palate so that saliva collects. Swallow the saliva.
4. **Massaging:** Rub both hands together to warm them; then massage them on the torso with downward movements from the solar plexus.
5. **Stretching:** Make your hands into fists and stretch your arms out from your body. Move them slowly back toward your body, using a pulling motion.
6. **Doubling:** Rest your fisted hands on your chest, and rotate the right shoulder forward, then the left. Rotate the right shoulder backward, then the left.
7. **Raising:** Raise the palms of your hand upward as you move your arms out. Bring the arms toward you with bent elbows until the palms are in front of your face. Work slowly and deliberately.
8. **Relaxing:** Sit on the floor, legs extended in front of you. Move your head forward while extending your arms toward your feet. Touch your toes if possible, without straining. Release; return to sitting with head upright.

Embryonic Breathing

One of the more fascinating meditative practices of the Taoist path is *T'ai Hsi* ("embryonic breathing"). It combines breathing meditation (identical to Yogic *pranayama*) with alchemical visualizations to extend life and dispel disease. As the name implies, it is a way of emulating the breathing pattern of the embryo. Training is required for this, because it is essential to learn the proper way to hold the breath and direct it to circulate through the complex of channels in the body.

A basic exercise to develop embryonic breathing is the visualization of *ch'i* entering the cinnabar fields and vitalizing them:

1. Begin in standing position, at the yang cycle of the day.
2. Consciously take in three normal breaths.
3. Take in the fourth breath and pause for a moment.
4. In this brief pause, see the air vitalize the lower cinnabar field. It goes through your nose to the navel, and it continues downward to your feet. Release the breath.
5. Take in the fifth breath and pause for a moment.
6. In this brief pause, see the air vitalize the middle cinnabar field. It goes from your nose to your spine. Release the breath.
7. Take in the sixth breath and pause for a moment.
8. In this brief pause, see the air vitalize the upper cinnabar field. It goes from your nose upward to the crown of your head.

As you repeat this exercise, you may feel different sensations in the cinnabar fields. This may be due to your inexperience in observing those regions of the body as you breathe. They have always been there, but your attention has not.

Feng Shui

Many of China's ancient arts have found their way to the West and made a significant impact on modern trends. One of them is *feng shui,* the art and science of creating a harmonious environment. It is grounded in the Taoist belief in *ch'i* and its effect on spaces, especially those created and inhabited by human beings.

Meditation aims to create a harmonious environment, and *feng shui* principles can aid in that process. The following sections cover some points that you may want to consider for your meditation oasis.

Sitting Space

This should be in an open area rather than a corner. An important consideration is the location of plumbing pipes and electrical wires. Whether they are overhead or beneath the floor, they should not be in the path of the sitting area. They are believed to divert the *ch'i* that meditation brings away from the practitioner.

Corners

These are areas where *ch'i* can be caught and stagnate. The introduction of living objects, such as flower arrangements or plants, can alleviate this tendency.

Areas Facing Traffic

Whether it is outside noise or household members passing by the room, this can disturb the *ch'i* that is generated in meditation. A table-sized water fountain can neutralize this, as well as encourage beneficial *ch'i* to anyone who enters.

Adjoining Rooms

The meditation space should not be passed through to reach an adjoining room. This will dissipate the efforts of the meditator and prevent progress.

Mirrors

Mirrors strategically placed can invite good influences and banish negative ones. Placing the *Pa Kua* before windows will draw beneficial influences into the room and balance the *ch'i* within. You can find small mirrors with the *Pa Kua* inscribed around the border in Asian stores and in many shops in the Chinatown districts of large cities.

Colors

Colors have a significant impact on the ambiance of the space. Each color is associated with one of the five elements and should be used accordingly:

Direction	Element	Color	Animal	Meaning
East	Wood	Blue, green	Dragon	Life, beginnings
West	Metal	White	Tiger	Death, endings
North	Water	Black	Tortoise	Calm, submission
South	Fire	Red	Phoenix	Strength, aggression
Center	Earth	Yellow	Meditator	Proliferation, stability

T'ai Chi: Grounding and Transforming

You may be familiar with the art of *t'ai chi,* because it has become a very popular form of exercise in the West. Its ability to bring relaxation to the mind and vitality to the body is well touted. In television and films about China, you will inevitably see individuals and groups practicing *t'ai chi* everywhere, at any time of day. They appear to be moving slowly, making hand passes and body movements in graceful, deliberate motions.

ALERT

An experienced *t'ai chi* teacher will evaluate the student's physical abilities before commencing instruction. You don't have to meet any expected abilities, but you will be observed to first see how you are presently handling your *ch'i.*

T'ai chi is actually the physical aspect of the ancient science of *ch'i kung* ("working the energy") that was recommended by Lao Tzu. The latter is a metaphysical system that does have physical practices, but it emphasizes the energetic aspect of the body and working with those currents and rhythms. *T'ai chi,* on the other hand, emphasizes relaxation through gentle movement. Its aim is to ground the body through exercises that make the meditator aware of the pulses of yin and yang, within and without. Through specific exercises that emulate natural forces—animals, plants, and elements like the wind—*ch'i* is also transformed. This is an important part of the practice, because it enhances both the mind and the life force.

While it is best to consult a teacher before you begin a practice, there are two exercises that can prepare you for the experience.

Finding Balance

Stand upright, feet slightly spaced with your dominant foot about four inches in front of the other. Balance yourself in this position.

Bend the knees slightly and start to rock, forward and backward. Movement should be very slow and deliberate, but do not press your feet into the floor. Your motions should be easy and subtle, as if you are surfing over water.

After rocking for two to three minutes, return to an upright standing posture and change your foot position. This time, the opposite foot will be placed in front of the dominant one. Repeat the forward-backward rocking motion with bent knees for two to three minutes.

Pay attention to any differences in your sensations of balance. Adjust your body stance accordingly when you repeat the exercise.

Finding the Center of Gravity

Stand upright, feet slightly spaced and evenly apart. Place your hands in front of your torso, palms facing inward but not touching your body.

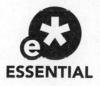

ESSENTIAL

Your center of gravity is the starting point for all *t'ai chi* exercises. In meditation, placing your hands over this center and resting them there provides inner balance. When you are feeling unwell, heat placed on this center can bring relief.

Begin conscious breathing, and as you do so, raise your palms upward as you inhale. Stop at the level of your lungs. On exhaling, lower your hands as far as they will go without bending. Repeat this slowly, for about three minutes. While breathing, focus your eyes on your hands, observing their movement up and down. Make note of any reactions in your hands as they pass over your torso.

You will notice an area in your torso where your hands are more sensitive and may react differently than at other areas. This is an indication of the center of the body's gravity. It may be above or below the navel, and either positioned on the right or the left.

Chinese Buddhism

The Buddhist stream made its way to China almost immediately following the passing of the Buddha. There, it mingled with existing traditions to create a number of specialty schools of Buddhism. For example, when fused with the mystical approach of Taoism, it created Ch'an ("meditation"), a very influential school that was introduced by a legendary figure, Bodhidharma, in the sixth century.

Some of the Buddhist doctrines were adapted to the established cultural mores, especially those that stemmed from the time-honored customs of Confucianism. For example, the regard for family life and ancestral reverence was central to Chinese society, and Buddhist practice adapted to that concept. As a result, long-dead Buddhist masters are revered as spiritual mentors in the same way that ancestors are viewed as helpful spirits to the living.

Taoism also exalted the innate powers of the natural world—in the skies, winds, and bodies of water. Buddhist practice adapted to that approach, placing meditation in nature as an ideal. China's arts and sciences—calligraphy, architecture, and medicine—also came to reflect this approach.

In Ch'an Buddhism, the process of enlightenment is described as "breaking through the three passes." The scholar Kulapati Yuan Ming of the Ching Dynasty described the "three passes" as follows:

- **The first pass:** The physical body must be realized as a mere combination of the four essential elements. This is to die "a great death" and to completely sweep away all illusions.
- **The second pass:** The ego must be identified with all things. This brings perfect compatibility between matter and emptiness. Then, utter freedom of the spirit is experienced.
- **The final pass:** Subjectivity and objectivity, meditator and meditated, substance and function must all become one. Then, blind desire and attachment fall away of their own accord.

Ch'an was the first to espouse an approach that was to have great impact on the practice of Buddhism in the following centuries and in countries where it later spread. Its emphasis on simplicity and its movement away from ritual attracted many. In Japan Ch'an reached its final flowering, transforming into Zen.

FACT

Falun Gong is derived from the science of Ch'i Kung, the mother lode of Taoist metaphysics. This practice views the body as a miniature universe. As such, it possesses all remedies for healing and all wisdom for self-knowledge. Entry into this universe and participation with its powers is the great treasure of the practice. That is why it poses such a threat to the temporal powers of communism.

Today, China is one of the last surviving communist countries, and certainly the largest. Yet despite nearly a century of religious oppression, many of the ancient practices of Taoism and Buddhism have persisted. In the late twentieth century especially, practitioners of Falun Gong ("Law Wheel energy cultivation"), an underground meditation movement, have faced grave dangers. Reliable reports have reached the West of some practitioners who, having gathered in groups to share their interests, were kidnapped and executed for their beliefs. Adherents of Falun Gong are said to number in the millions.

CHAPTER 12

The Art of Listening

There once was a time when only the sounds of nature could be heard around the world. The noises of civilization were few, and far less intrusive than today. Human beings have adapted in many ways to the harmful sounds of industry and technology. In the process, we have considerably diminished our capacity for awareness.

Becoming Totally Aware

Have you ever seen a cat sleeping? It's not difficult, since they're asleep most of the time, or so we believe. In deep repose, they are apparently oblivious to everything in the waking world. But rattle a box of catnip, or unwrap the cellophane around a fish fillet, and they are not only awake, but fully alert.

Catnapping is an example of how both complete rest and total awareness are possible, at least in the animal world. But some meditative approaches recognize this state of mind as a distinct possibility for human beings, too.

The Zen Tradition

The term Zen is the Japanese translation of Ch'an, the Chinese school of Mahayana Buddhism that reached Japan in the twelfth century. Ch'an is itself the Chinese transcription of the Sanskrit *Dyana* ("meditation"). Ch'an appeared with the legendary figure of Bodhidharma, who came from India in the sixth century to teach Buddhism in Canton, China. He was a rascally character, and bizarre stories are told of his unconventional behavior and teachings. It's said that he sat for seven years facing the wall in meditation at the Shao-lin monastery. Bodhidharma's approach was "direct, to the mind, and without words." He also pointed out that Buddhahood could be achieved by fully discovering one's true nature.

As the Buddhist tradition was transmitted from China to Japan, many branches flourished. The first major school to take root was the Tendai in the seventh century. It was based on the study of Buddhist philosophy and writings, especially the Lotus Sutra. This was believed to be the highest teaching and expression of the enlightened Buddha. Another school arose shortly afterward, the Shingon. Instead of emphasizing the scholarly and contemplative practice of the Tendai, the Shingon gravitated toward a mystical approach. As in the Tantric practices of Tibet, it made great use of the mandala, the mudra, and mantra.

In 1200, at age fourteen, a young man named Eihei Dogen entered a Tendai monastery. But by age twenty-three, he sought other ways to discover self-knowledge. With one of his teachers, he journeyed to China to study Ch'an, seeking the most authentic form of Buddhism. It was there that he discovered *zazen* ("sitting"), the style of meditation that emulates the Buddha's approach. On returning to Japan, he was charged by his teachers to propagate this teaching.

ESSENTIAL

The middle way emphasizes the approach that the Buddha employed to accomplish the supreme goal: meditation. In Japan, it is *zazen*, which simply means "sitting."

The rise of Zen took place at a critical time in Japanese history. It was concurrent with the establishment of the Shogunate, rulers who came from the samurai ("warrior") class. They were not particularly drawn to either the rituals of Shingon or the studies of Tendai. Instead, they found a practical approach to mental and spiritual development in Zen. It was "direct, to the mind, and without words." Over time, it even offered some physical approaches that could be applied to the warrior arts.

The Meditating Buddha

Zen teachers point out that the Buddha's experiences are the essential guideposts for enlightenment. He began life as a prince, living in great luxury that sheltered him from any experience of hardship. He then began his spiritual journey. To reach stillness of the body and emotions, Siddhartha underwent extreme austerity, relinquishing food, drink, and all the comforts of everyday existence. He followed the path of the ancient *sannyasin* (ascetic), but it did not contribute to his self-knowledge. Instead, he realized that a "middle way" was the path to enlightenment. Having everything did not bring it, nor did the mortification of the flesh. This middle way is the central theme in Buddhism, and especially in Zen. Because when all is said and done, the experience of inner enlightenment will only make a difference if it enriches the individual's life in the outer world.

Zen Sitting Accessories

Zen meditation is simple, but getting started with some helpful accessories is essential. The Japanese are experts in the design of meditation environments. Here are some of the items that you might incorporate to create a comfortable meditation oasis in the Zen style:

- **Futon ("mattress"):** Usually a large, flat, cotton-stuffed pad used for sitting or sleeping.
- **Zabuton ("sitting mat"):** A traditionally dark blue woven mat or pad that is placed on a flat surface prior to meditation.
- **Zafu ("sitting cushion"):** A small, round black pillow placed over the *zabuton*. When sitting, it is centered under the buttocks to create an imaginary triangle with the *zafu* at one corner and each of the folded knees touching the remaining corners.

FACT

In Zen meditation, the hands rest at the navel, which the Japanese call *hara*. It is regarded as the balancing point in the body, the hub of gravity. It is also viewed as the core of the life force and the center of the universe.

Zen Teachings

Two approaches to Zen practice evolved, reflecting the old Tendai and Shingon approaches.

Rinzai School

Purposeful and disciplined, Rinzai reflects the samurai virtues of detachment, self-discipline, and complete awareness of the moment. One of its teachings is the *Shi-ryoken* ("four ways of seeing"). It is a philosophy that demonstrates the progression from ordinary to enlightened existence:

- There can be no subject without an object.
- The external world is a projection of the individual's conscious mind.

- There is a state of consciousness where subject and object are transcended.
- There is no subject and object.

Rinzai emphasizes the *koans*. These are written or spoken riddles that become a mental enigma, and are used as a device for meditation. Human beings are restrained by the straitjacket of language and concepts. Because the *koan* departs from logical processes, it becomes a vehicle for leaving ordinary thinking and entering the vibrant world of the Buddha mind. The *koan* may be a teaching, a realization, or an event in the life of a teacher.

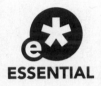

ESSENTIAL

Koans for contemplation include the following: What was the face you had before you were born? The flag doesn't move, only your mind moves. What is the sound of one hand clapping? From where you are, stop the distant boat from moving across the water. Who is it that hears?

Another approach to the *koan* is to ask yourself, while becoming aware of any activity, who is experiencing that activity. For example, when eating, ask, "Who is eating?" When walking, ask, "Who is walking?"

Soto School

The school of Dogen is simple and direct, reflecting the natural approach to enlightenment. There is an emphasis on *shikantaza* ("nothing but sitting"), with *zazen* as the central practice. As simple as this sounds, it must involve all aspects of the meditator. The mind is free of thought, but there is also a "razor's edge" state of mind that is cultivated, where there are no distractions. Counting the breath and meditation upon *koans* is rejected in favor of "sitting as the Buddha sat."

The differences between the Rinzai and the Soto schools are subtle to some, but they suit different personality types. The Rinzai is likened to "the frost of late autumn," while the Soto is compared to "the spring breeze that caresses the flower."

The Monkey Mind

Zen teachings speak considerably about the mind: its tendency to wander, run a habitual course, and become absorbed. It is referred to as the monkey mind, because like a monkey it jumps from branch to branch.

FACT

The Buddhism that is found in Japan is fused, as it has been in other Asian cultures, with the indigenous religion. Shinto ("way of the gods") existed until the nineteenth century as Japan's dominant spiritual practice, but Buddhist thought superseded Shinto with the onset of the industrial age. Still, many concepts and deities particular to its culture have remained in the practice of Japanese Buddhist meditation.

The activity of the mind is, paradoxically, "mindless." There is, however, more to the dimension of mind than this activity. And that's what Zen meditation is meant to enter. There are several approaches:

- **Attention:** Becoming aware of the mind's activity. It is possible to detach from thoughts by viewing them, as each passes by. Pay attention to the mind.
- **Visualization:** There are some "countering" techniques that can be used to slow the mind's moving from thought to thought. Visual scenes, seed thoughts, everyday objects, and actions are all employed. They may be in the immediate environment or mentally evoked.
- **Focus:** Each time the mind wanders from a visualization, it is brought back. Naturally, this goes back to developing attention and visualization, but one must be gentle in the process, and not force or concentrate the mind.
- **Quieting:** The senses are quieted to achieve and maintain focus. This may entail entering a serene environment in which all stimulation is minimal and reflects a theme of serenity.

The Ten Fetters

In Zen, there are cautions that remind the meditator to clear the mind and maintain stillness. These are the ten fetters, which constrain the mind from reaching stillness:

1. **The ego:** It is the ego of personality that creates illusion. Of course, the ego is a vehicle for our identity, but only in the temporal world. In the world of true reality, there is no ego.
2. **Skepticism:** The mind accepts and rejects at will. This prevents inquiry and the progressive discovery of truth.
3. **Attachment to ritual:** Despite the value of daily and religious rituals, they can hinder the understanding of eternal principles.
4. **The senses:** These are often the vehicle for delusion of what is beneficial and what is not.
5. **Ill will:** Emotions that block acceptance of self and others prevent well-being of body and mind.
6. **Materialism:** Dependence on tangible things diverts our energies to meaningless thoughts and actions.
7. **Desire for an immaterial life:** Even the search for spirituality can become a fetter, when it fails to enrich our involvement with the outer world.
8. **Arrogance:** The belief that one has accomplished more than others or that one has attained perfect knowledge is erroneous.
9. **Restlessness:** This leads to the wandering mind and the inability to focus attention.
10. **Ignorance of the true nature of reality:** This is the condition of most human beings, and is the reason for practicing *zazen*.

The Ten Perfections

There are also bywords to remind the meditator of conditions that should be cultivated in order to reach enlightenment:

1. **Generosity:** The belief that all that is surrendered is eventually returned, perhaps in another form, but in the most beneficial way.
2. **Morality:** Ethical conduct leads to respect of self and others.

3. **Renunciation:** The material life can only lead so far on the journey to enlightenment.
4. **Wisdom:** We never know whether we are wise or not, but the choice of wise action is always available to us.
5. **Energy:** Life endows us with boundless energy to discover truth and the nature of reality.
6. **Patience:** We must be patient above all with ourselves. This patience is extended to those around us when we accept that all events happen in their own time and place, not ours.
7. **Truthfulness:** This becomes possible when we are dedicated to knowing truth ourselves.
8. **Resolution:** We are only able to accomplish when our resolve is centered in every act we undertake. Then, failure is not possible.
9. **Lovingkindness:** These two words become one when we maintain an accepting attitude toward ourselves and others.
10. **Calm mind:** No matter what events or feelings arise, the cultivation and maintenance of stillness brings calm to ourselves and to everything around us.

ESSENTIAL

In Zen, the mind is likened to a still body of water. Thoughts are like clouds that pass overhead. They are reflected in the water, but they are not in it. Likewise, the senses are like ripples in the water that come from the activity of feeling. They, too, pass by.

Listening Meditation

An important approach to meditation in the Zen style can be described in one word: listening. And this does not mean simply hearing with the ears. It means listening with one's entire being.

Start with the sitting posture and relax your body through breathing. You may count your breaths, from one to ten, then start over again. This is a typical approach to monitoring the breath and focusing the mind in *zazen*, but it's optional.

You may close your eyes to maintain focus, but remember that Zen meditation calls for focusing all the senses. You will open your eyes after a degree of mental stillness is achieved.

FACT

After all is said and done, Zen philosophy reminds us that the real world awaits our attention. In a most pragmatic manner, this branch of Buddhism has emphasized that the meditator should express the serenity and insight brought by meditation in his surroundings.

Listen attentively, for about five minutes. Do not try to identify the sounds, or where they come from. Listen only to the sounds. Then, open your eyes. Listen attentively again with your eyes open, five more minutes.

Zen Art

Zen art and creativity meshed with the written Japanese language through standards of design and calligraphy. Environmentally, disciplines arose for flower arranging, the design and function of dwellings and garden, and social customs such as the tea ceremony. The marvel of these activities is that they have become vehicles for meditation itself.

In Japanese culture, daily contact with nature is valued as an essential way to maintain mental and physical health. One art that embodies this dictate is *kado* ("the way of flowers"). Like other Zen-influenced arts, *kado* is a way to enhance or bring out the innate beauty and simplicity in the environment. It is an approach to unlocking and experiencing the purity of things around us. The process of doing this is part of the meditation; experiencing it is the other part.

Another idea that is incorporated in Zen art is the principle of spontaneity arising from controlled conditions. In other words, what we expect to happen is not necessarily going to happen. It may be something altogether different, and surprising, and beautiful in its uniqueness. This is what is sought in *sumiye,* the art of calligraphy. Following a prescribed ritual of mixing the inks, preparing the paper, and holding the brush in traditional ways, the inscription of letters can come out amazingly pure and natural.

A Zen Tea Break

The Japanese tea ceremony *Cha-no Yu* ("water for tea") was originally devised to prevent monks from falling asleep during deep meditation exercise. Gradually, the discipline itself became a ritualized ceremony, providing an opportunity for the contemplation of timeless images. And with the ceremony arose the art of constructing the teahouse, as well as crafting accessories, such as the cups and water pots, furniture, even the brooms for sweeping. Of themselves they also became ritualized productions, providing additional approaches to the meditation experience.

QUOTE

> We cover fragile bones
> In their festive best
> To view
> Immortal flowers.
>
> —Matsuo Basho, seventeenth-century Japanese poet

Although the tea ceremony is a group meditation, you may observe it on your own. A separate space is ideal for this, where fresh flowers, a tidy table, and a comfortable chair can be placed. Traditionally, the ceremony is held in the teahouse, with the participants sitting on the floor on a *tatami* mat and cushions. The ceremony is quite elaborate, and dictated by a protocol that covers every possible detail. The manner of entering the room, sitting, and speaking are outlined with guidelines of simplicity and flawlessness.

Zen Tea
Container of cold water
Powdered or loose green tea with a scoop
Strainer for the tea and a dish to place it in

Start the fire. Pour the water slowly and deliberately into the heating container and place it on the fire. Watch the water as it heats. When it comes to a rolling boil, remove it from the fire and scoop the tea into it. Cover and allow it to steep for a few minutes. Pour the tea into a teapot, using the strainer.

Drinking the Tea

Drinking the tea isn't as simple as it sounds. Observe the following steps:

1. Pour the tea into a cup.
2. Pick up the cup with your right hand and place it in the left hand, with the fingers of the right hand still around the cup. Your thumb should be facing you. Make a small, polite bow.
3. Now, turn the bowl clockwise 90 degrees with the thumb and forefinger of your right hand. Take a sip, and allow the fragrance of the tea to rise up to your nose.
4. Finish drinking the tea in small sips. When you are finished, inhale deeply and audibly.
5. Turn the cup counterclockwise 90 degrees with the thumb and forefinger back to its original position when you picked it up.

The focus of *Cha-no Yu* is always the tea. Zen points to focusing attention in the moment, toward the essentials of the here-and-now. In the tea ceremony, the anticipation, preparation, and enjoyment of the tea conveys the sense of timelessness and focused awareness.

The Language of Zen

Most of the terms used in Zen practice are Japanese translations of Buddhist concepts taken from the original Sanskrit. This knowledge arrived in Japan via Korea in the sixth century. Important terms include:

- **Dojo:** The place of teaching, where students meet for instruction
- **Kensho:** The Zen equivalent of nirvana, the state of enlightenment—a rare and momentary attainment
- **Roshi:** A Zen master, equivalent to the guru
- **Satori:** The Zen concept of the enlightened state, a profound awakening that is reached spontaneously, though it is a transitory condition
- **Sensei:** The Zen teacher, used in address as well as name
- **Zazen ("sitting"):** The act of meditation

Reiki and Johrei

Zen is a practice that has moved away from ritual, religion, and philosophy. In many meditation circles, Zen is no longer associated with Buddhism and has become a model for beneficial psychoanalytic solutions to modern problems. Moreover, it has given rise to other systems that promote the restoration of health on other levels.

In the nineteenth century, the Japanese theologian Dr. Mikao Usui received a powerful revelation through meditation. In it, he perceived that the miraculous healing techniques of Jesus and the Buddha were not only similar; others could know them as well. One of his students, Chujiro Hayashi, organized the vision into a methodology that today has thousands of adherents.

Reiki (*rei,* "universal," and *ki,* "life force") is a system of developing and enhancing healing energy. After this is accomplished, certain hand postures are practiced to heal oneself and others. The chakras are key points in the system, and developing a sensitive awareness of body energy is important. In modern times, it is taught in three stages or levels.

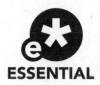

ESSENTIAL

Some might view these practices as forms of "psychic" healing, or the laying on of hands, but many physicians are now looking at these techniques seriously. Alternative medicine is still in its infancy in the West, while the Orient has practiced it for centuries. These approaches, along with meditation, are offering viable ways of restoring the well-being in body and mind through connecting with spirit.

Johrei ("spirit purification") is another energy-related healing technique derived from the Japanese application of Buddhist philosophy to health. It involves the focused invocation of healing energy that is transferred to the patient. In both Reiki and Johrei, the practitioner must engage in extended meditation exercises and techniques. The practitioner must become "healed" before becoming a healer, and that involves going to the source of healing, the universal life force. Some see the universal life force as divine energy or light, but the premise is the same. It exists, and it may be experienced, enhanced, and given to those in need.

CHAPTER 13

Poetic Inspiration

Some words can steer us into high regions of thought and feeling. Aside from expressing ideas, they can also be stepping stones that create pathways to understanding profound mysteries. Poets know this, and they take us on such journeys in moments of quiet reflection.

The Islamic Tradition

Combined with movement, words are keys to liberating us from the ordinary world. Nearly every culture has developed this kind of expression, and comparing the common threads that run through the traditions is a fascinating study. Words of wisdom and insight are passed down through generations, telling the same story, though perhaps in different ways. Melodies may accompany them, along with gestures that have special meaning. The oral heritage is a respected approach to self-knowledge, because it encourages the listener to reflect on the meaning, based on her experience.

Islam (which means "submission") is a religious practice that espouses submission of the individual will to the will of the Creator. Most Muslims (practitioners of the Islamic religion) live in an area that encompasses a wide swath over half of the planet, from Africa to the Middle East, and continuing to Asia and the South Pacific.

FACT

Sufism has acquired a meaning that departs from religious connotations. Instead, it indicates a mystical or occult approach to spiritual experience. In most Islamic countries, a mystical seeker is now regarded as a Sufi no matter what his country of origin or religious persuasion. It has come to denote a state of being that emphasizes a unity the practitioner feels with others and with God.

The Sunni and the Shi'ah

Two main groups comprise this tradition: the Sunni and the Shi'ah. The largest group of Muslims (85 percent as of the year 2000) is the Sunni; most live in West Africa, Egypt, Palestine, Turkey, Syria, Saudi Arabia, and Afghanistan. The Wahhabi, a prominent subgroup, live primarily in Saudi Arabia. The Sunni consider their following to stem from Fatima, the daughter of Muhammad and his only immediate descendant. The minority group is the Shi'ah; most of its followers live in Iran and the remaining live in Iraq, Lebanon, and Bahrain. The Shi'ah consider their following to stem from Ali, who was Muhammad's son-in-law.

In the first century following the Hegira, or flight of Mohammed from Mecca to Medina in 622, a small group arose called the Sufis. Their name is derived from the Arabic *suf* ("wool") because they wore white woolen robes. The movement came into being as a reaction against the warrior cult of the Umayyads. The Sufis chose a mystical path and moved toward an esoteric interpretation of Islam.

ESSENTIAL

The Qu'ran is the holy book that was given to the prophet Muhammad by the archangel Gabriel, following an extended period of meditation and asceticism in a cave near Mecca.

The Five Pillars of Islam

In Islam, divine law is presented in the Qu'ran ("the reading"). In the Qu'ran, *Suras* ("chapters") present mystical concepts and a historical record of the human race. However, in essence, the Qu'ran is a guide to living in oneness with God and with others in compassion and forgiveness. The Five Pillars, or fundamental precepts, are the basis of this guide:

1. **Shahadah ("the affirmation of faith"):** There is no god but God and Muhammad is his prophet.
2. **Salat ("the five prayers"):** Offered at dawn, midday, midafternoon, sunset, and at night by all adult male and female Muslims, these prayers are said following ritual ablutions and always on Friday, the Lord's Day.
3. **Sawam ("observance of Ramadan"):** From the time of puberty, all Muslims abstain from food, drink, sex, and tobacco, from dawn until sunset, during the ninth holy lunar month of Ramadan.
4. **Zakat ("offering of alms"):** The faithful share wealth through assisting the poor and orphans, which purifies the donor from greed and stinginess.
5. **Hajj ("pilgrimage"):** This journey to Mecca, the holy seat of Islam, must be made at least once in the lifetime of the practitioner.

The Sufi Experience

Though it may appear at first glance that the Sufi pathway is more spontaneous than prescribed, there is a science of achieving the unity with God that is the central aim of the practice. It is outlined in three stages:

1. **Sair ita Allah:** Progress toward God, which leads to *fana*
2. **Sair fi Allah:** Progress within God; the experience of divine unity, and acquiring divine attributes in the process, which is *baqa*
3. **Sair 'ani Allah:** Progress beyond God; attainment of nonexistence, the permanent state of *fana*

The third stage cannot be approached through study or teachings. It can only be approached through direct experience, which has four components:

1. **Dhikr:** Chanting the name of God
2. **Riyadat:** Ascetic practices such as fasting
3. **Inkisar:** Detachment from worldly things and conditions
4. **Subha:** Surrendering the ego to the absolute reality

The poet Rumi advocated the calling of the divine name as the supreme approach to awakening the divine presence within. In the Sufi tradition, this is performed in conjunction with rhythmic breathing.

Five Purification Breaths

The exercise that prepares the practitioner for rhythmic breathing is the five purifications of the soul. The universal elements are the focal points, being earth, water, fire, and air. Begin at sunrise if possible, when the elements are at their peak. Stand upright.

Breathe slowly and deeply, keeping in mind the energy of the earth. Visualize it as the color yellow, entering your body as you inhale through the nose. The earth element travels upward from the ground through your spine to your crown. As it does so, the earth filters out all impurities. It returns to the ground when you exhale through the nose. Repeat this four more times.

Breathe slowly and deeply, keeping in mind the energy of water. Visualize it as the color green, entering your nose as you inhale. The water element moves upward from the stomach, through your spine to your crown. As it does so, the liquid washes away all impurities. It exits from your stomach when you exhale through the mouth. Repeat this four more times.

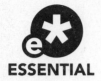

ESSENTIAL

Following the breathing purifications, recite the divine name. In Islam, the names of God are manifold, but there is only one God. This dictate is cited in the Qu'ran and becomes the Sufi mantra for awakening the divine presence within: (*La ilaha illa-llah: Mohammedan rasul Al-lah.*) "There is no God but God: and Muhammad is his prophet."

Breathe slowly and deeply, keeping in mind the energy of fire. Visualize it as the color red, entering your body through your heart as you inhale. The fire element moves upward to your crown. As it does so, the fire burns away all impurities. It exits from your heart when you exhale through the nose. Repeat this four times (a total of five).

Breathe slowly and deeply, keeping in mind the energy of air. Visualize it as the color blue, entering your body through all of your pores as you inhale. The air element moves through all the organs and tissues, blowing away all the impurities. It exits through the pores when you exhale through your mouth. Repeat this four times (a total of five).

Direct Experience

Sufism is an expression similar to Bhakti Yoga, the experience of seeing the divine presence in everything and honoring that divinity. There is simplicity in this approach, along with a rich and resonant love that transcends (but also includes) the personal realm. However, the Sufis depart from the Bhakti Yoga tradition in that they do not revere gurus or teachers. Rather, they seek truth within themselves. Only angels can guide them.

In the West, Sufi dancing has drawn considerable interest. There is some hesitation, however, for women to participate due to the traditionally segregated nature of Islam. Even though women played a significant role in the life of Muhammad, prevailing customs keep much of the practice separated for men and women.

Ecstatic Dance

Unless you are a member of a Sufi *tariqa*, the modern experience of Sufism is limited to viewing dervish performances in theaters and events in some Muslim countries. Participation by outsiders is limited, although spiritual pilgrims are always welcomed. In the West, a movement called Dances of Universal Peace was established in the 1960s to explore Sufi dancing as a meditative art form.

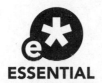

ESSENTIAL

Hadith is the narrative record of the Qu'ran that explains its precepts and provides commentary. *Taqwa* is God consciousness, which is endowed to every human being. *Tasawwuf* is the true name of the mystical path known as Sufism.

The program of Dances of Universal Peace seeks to unite participants of all religious persuasions in the experience of sacred dance. A typical gathering begins with a rhythmic walking meditation in a circle to unify the participants in mind. Then, music accompanies simple dances around the circle. There is an emphasis on meeting with each person in the circle through turning and greeting. This is an important aspect of acknowledging the oneness of all present.

Mantras or phrases of sacred names are also incorporated in the modern Sufi dances. There are recitations of the many words for God: Allah, Yeshua (Jesus), Buddha, and Rama (among many others). The recitations are chanted to the rhythm of the music.

Many nondenominational groups around the world now sponsor Dances of Universal Peace on a recurring basis. There are local chapters in some major U.S. cities, and events are held at Unitarian churches and on university campuses.

The Sikhs

In the fifteenth century, a religious teacher in what is now Pakistan attempted to remedy the segregation of the sexes and classes in religious practice.

In addition, he also sought to reconcile the prevailing religions of his day: Islam, Hinduism, and Buddhism. Guru Nanak founded the Sikh ("disciple") movement, a mystical sect that practiced trance meditation and believed in one God and harmonious living.

FACT

Sacred dance is not a new idea, and many indigenous cultures use dance as a major component in their practices. The fusion of the senses with mind can allow the meditator to depart from ordinary consciousness and enter exalted states of mind and feeling.

Nanak wrote the *Jap-ji,* a collection of poems that is now the Sikh guiding principle. He spoke of union with the divine presence and methods by which it could be realized. His spiritual approach was a fusion of Bhakti and Tantra Yoga with Sufism. One of the mantras of the practice expresses this cohesion:

Eck Ong Kar Sat Nam Siri Wha Guru.
The Supreme is One, His names are many.

The Sikhs also recognize the elemental forces that Sufism presents, although they are associated with qualities of mind:

Earth teaches us patience and love;
Air teaches us mobility and liberty;
Fire teaches us warmth and courage;
Sky teaches us equality and broadmindedness;
Water teaches us purity and cleanliness.
We will imbibe these qualities in Nature
For our personalities to be fuller, happier, and nobler.

The Sikhs are distinguished by their uncut beards and hair, which they wear in elaborate turbans. They have a strict practice of cleanliness and courtesy, and are tolerant of all classes and religions. All men carry the surname of Singh ("lion") and the women are Kaur ("princess").

The Metaphysical Tradition

One of the modern exponents of esoteric Islam was the French scholar and mystic René Guénon. Born in 1886, he became interested in religion and occultism at an early age. He began a career of writing for scholarly journals on diverse subjects such as Hindu doctrine and the Christian mysteries. But in the process, he also initiated a journey of discovering the metaphysical basis of all traditions.

Guénon was a modern day gnostic ("seeker of revelation"). Beneath the tangle of the world's religions and mythologies, he sought the common underlying threads. His writing reflects those discoveries, and the meanings that those threads can convey to thoughtful seekers. A collection of those insights is found in *Fundamental Symbols: The Universal Language of Sacred Science*. In it, he discusses "eternal ideas," or universal themes that are found in all spiritual traditions. They include the well-recognized icons of the cross, the wheel, the Sun, and the four compass points.

QUOTE

"One who is absorbed in the Beloved and has renounced all else is a Sufi."
—Najm ad-Din Kubra (1145–1221), founder of the Kubrawiya Sufi brotherhood in Persia

The problems of Western civilization were also of great concern to Guénon. He believed that tradition had been abandoned, and materialism was creating a society of "man machines." In keeping with the path of the contemplative scholar, he took the name Abed el Wahed Yahia and moved to Egypt, where he lived until his death in 1951.

CHAPTER 14

The Power of Prayer

As the Eastern traditions brought mysticism and metaphysics to the West in the nineteenth and twentieth centuries, many seekers began to discover that there are more similarities than differences between their spiritual approaches. For example, prayer vigils in Western contemplative communities share many similarities to the meditation retreats of the East. This chapter begins with the premise that prayer and meditation are not two separate activities but part and parcel of the same inner phenomenon.

The Spiritual Ideal

Monastic traditions in the East and West share many features, among them the aspiration to emulate an ideal figure. Devotion to this ideal is expressed in the same way: surrender of the ego, or emptying oneself of personal thoughts and desires. Personal energies and attention are directed to the ideal, to knowing it fully and becoming part of it.

The Buddhists call on Avalokitesvara, the "regarder of the cries of the world" for spiritual aid. The Chinese know this divine being as Kwan Yin; the Hindus see him as Krishna; and the Japanese call him Kannon. Possessing boundless compassion and mercy, this exalted spirit walks on earth in many forms and places, responding to the immense suffering in human life that has begged for relief through the ages. Through all the recountings of their lives and works, these deliverers have a common theme, the union of the soul with the creative source, God.

Prayer is common in this pursuit, even though at first glance it may not seem so. Both Eastern and Western traditions seek the cultivation of silence as a meditative practice. Also, reflection on the qualities of the ideal figure, such as compassion and humility, is important. But what binds these practices together is a desire to allow the peace of meditative practice to enter everyday life.

The Teacher of Righteousness

Many mysteries surround the life and ministry of Jesus the Nazarene, born at the beginning of the Common Era in Bethlehem, Palestine. There are few details about his youth and education, but Jesus appeared at a critical time in Jewish history. Roman domination of the region had created immense hardship on its inhabitants. The Romans considered religious expression a threat to the supremacy of the Caesars, the emperors who had proclaimed themselves gods. All citizens of the Roman Empire were required to pay *obeisance* to the Caesars.

Jesus, a devout Jewish man, began a self-determined ministry at the age of thirty. At the time, there were several divisions in the Jewish faith. The orthodox Jews followed the strict dictates of the Sadducees, while the more liberal segment of society followed the Pharisees. A monastic tradition also existed. These followers, who lived separately in the region of the Dead Sea away from the great cities, pursued a contemplative, mystical approach to Judaism. Many scholars believe that Jesus was a member of this movement. The Dead Sea Scrolls, found in 1947, were the records of this community and reveal provocative details about their beliefs. Among other things, they cite a "teacher of righteousness" who is believed to be Jesus. His role was to reveal the mysteries locked in the Scriptures.

ESSENTIAL

The life and death of Jesus became the fountainhead of a religious movement that changed the face of Western civilization. His two exhortations are the cornerstones of Christian doctrine: to love God above all other things and to love your neighbor as you love yourself.

The Gnostics

In 1945, a cache of ancient papyrus scrolls was discovered in a remote region near Nag Hammadi, Egypt. After years of negotiating their ownership, scholars were able to determine that they dated from the fourth century. They were apparently copied from even older texts, by a community of Christian ascetics known at the time as Gnostics ("those who know"). The term is also used to denote "insight."

The early Christian church regarded the Gnostics as heretics because their gospels were unauthorized by the early Church. The Nag Hammadi scrolls are believed to be remnants of those gospels and their contents have surprised and mystified scholars. They include teachings on spiritual practice and statements that closely resemble Buddhist thought. Excerpts have been compared to Zen *koans.* In one statement, Christ says to one of his disciples:

If you bring forth what is in you,
What you bring forth will save you.
If you do not bring forth what is within you,
What you do not bring forth will destroy you.

Prayer or Meditation?

Meditation has always been labeled an Eastern tradition, while prayer is particular to the West. This is far from the truth, because both are essentially the same in spirit and practice. Here are some examples of what prayer and meditation share:

- Recognition of the connections among heart, mind, and spirit
- Realization that divine energy or grace exists in and around the world of life
- Cultivation of qualities of good character
- Discovery of a higher power through practice

In addition, the traditions that promote meditation or prayer offer a variety of approaches to unify heart, mind, and spirit, and they teach that divine energy or grace is accessible to us. It's not hard to see that the reasons for practicing them are shared by every spiritual path we've examined. Only dogma separates them.

But, you might ask, isn't prayer directed to a separate entity and meditation directed to the self? Actually, the writings of Christian theologians resemble the teachings of the other traditions in many ways. Most importantly, the path to the higher power lies through the efforts of the individual alone. Only the route is different.

If we were to compare the approaches of meditation and prayer as paths on the journey from conscious existence to superconscious experience, it is really very simple. Meditation employs the mind; prayer employs the heart.

The Monastic Tradition

One of the first early Christians to formally retreat from society was a young man named Macarius, who began an austere life in Wadi Natrun in the western desert of Egypt. By the fourth century, the dissolution of the Roman Empire was underway, and many sought the peace and serenity offered by religious life. By the time Macarius passed away at the age of ninety, more than 4,000 monks had been drawn to his monastery alone. The movement was so widespread that a century later, the daughter of the emperor Zeno joined the community disguised as a monk. After centuries of building, raids by a variety of rulers, and a renaissance in monastic life, the monastery of Macarius still flourishes today.

In the following centuries, those circumstances were repeated throughout the Mediterranean. From Egypt and the Sinai to Greece, and westward to Europe, all classes of people joined spiritual communities to contemplate the life of Christ and practice his two exhortations.

FACT

> Monks (from the Greek *monos,* meaning "alone") initially lived in caves at the extremity of civilization. Their initial goal was threefold: to reach *apatheia* ("pacification"), where the passions are quieted; to practice *hesychia* ("reposing in silence"), where the mind withdraws from the outer world to reflect on spiritual realities; and to attain *metanoia* ("all being together"), where the soul is transformed.

Monastic life followed a rule of order that dictated every daily activity. Prayer was the central practice throughout the day, punctuated only by domestic duties assigned to each member. Reflective time was also allotted to the study of Scripture to provide inspiration. Guidelines were established that included poverty, chastity, and obedience. And like the Buddhist monasteries, those of the Middle Ages "specialized" with a particular approach to emulating the life of Christ. Some were dedicated to healing the sick, others to teaching or preserving Christian writings.

The Contemplatives

Over time, withdrawal from the outside world became more than an accepted way to exercise the contemplative side of Christianity. The life of seclusion evolved into one of the few ways to receive an education or practice the arts. Gradually, those realms became intertwined with monastic life, so much so that the artistic and intellectual legacy of Western culture is innately connected to its spiritual tradition. The contemplative life encouraged this, and it is being revived today to encourage creative people to unlock their potential.

Conditions in the eleventh century brought these circumstances to a summit. In 1098, Hildegard of Bingen was born to a noble family in what is now Germany. From childhood she appeared to be unworldly, and she entered the religious life at fifteen. Until the age of forty-two, she pursued the contemplative regimen of the convent. Then she reported a revelatory vision, in which she understood "the meaning of the expositions of the books . . . the evangelists and other catholic books of the Old and New Testaments." More importantly, she also saw that her future work was to write and expound what she understood in her revelation.

The work and writings of Hildegard reflect that this revelation was more than an intuitive flash. She produced extensive theological works on Christian doctrine, poetry, music, morality plays, and scientific works on botany and medicine. She also presented a supremely meditative view on interpreting the Gospel of St. John. Seeing it as an allegory of the spiritual condition of the human race, she urged contemplation on spiritual rather than literal meanings of the Scriptures in her public teaching.

Hildegard did not go about her life quietly in a plain nun's habit, praying and contemplating throughout the day. Until her passing in 1179, she conducted herself as a resourceful manager of a convent, a composer, teacher, and artist. She is said to have worn colorful clothes and appreciated beautiful gems and scents. She was regarded by her peers as prophetic and saw profoundly into the mystical dimension of nature. Hildegard wrote:

The earth is at the same time mother,
She is mother of all that is natural, mother of all that is human.
She is the mother of all, for contained in her are the seeds of all.
The earth of humankind contains all moistness, all verdancy,
All germinating power.
It is in so many ways fruitful.
All creation comes from it.
Yet it forms not only the basic raw material for mankind,
But also the substance of the incarnation of God's son.

The Revelation of St. Francis of Assisi

In the thirteenth century, despite an early life of privilege and ease, a young Italian named Francesco di Bernadone received a spiritual command through prayer to dedicate his life to peace and contemplation. In answer to this, he was to found the brotherhood of the "little friars." They came to play a significant role in European spirituality in the following centuries as the Franciscans.

A former knight, Francesco began a new life in Assisi to live in imitation and union with Christ. Besides preaching and cultivating an attitude of complete equanimity with men and nature, he lived in complete poverty. When critics of the church admonished him, he argued that he was truly free.

He did not see the tangible world as separate from divine life. Rather, he recognized nature as both a gift and a reflection of God that gives beauty and usefulness to humanity. His writings reflect these views powerfully. In one of his well-known prayers, the five elements and the luminaries are intertwined in his perception of this radiant world:

Praised be you my Lord, with all your creatures,
Especially my Lord Brother Sun,
Who brings the day, and by whom you enlighten us.
He is beautiful, he shines with great splendor;
Of you, Most High, he is the symbol.
Praised be you, my Lord, for Sister Moon and the stars,
In the heavens you formed them clear, precious, and beautiful.
Praised be you, my Lord, for Brother Wind and for the air and for the clouds,
For the azure calm and for all climes by which you give life to your creatures.
Praised be you, my Lord, for Sister Water
Who is very useful and humble, humble and chaste.
Praised be you, my Lord, for Brother Fire,
By whom you enlighten the night.
He is beautiful and joyous, indomitable and strong.
Praised be you, my Lord, for our Mother the Earth
Who nourishes us and bears us, and produces all kinds of fruits,
With the speckled flowers and the herbs.

On his deathbed in 1226, it is reported that St. Francis repeated a last addition to this prayer: "Praised be you, my Lord, for our Sister Death."

St. Francis of Assisi wrote the following meditation on peace:

Lord, make me an instrument of your peace;
Where there is hatred, let me sow love;
Where there is injury, pardon;
Where there is doubt, faith;
Where there is despair, hope;
Where there is darkness, light;
And where there is sadness, joy.
Grant that I may not so much seek to be consoled as to console;
To be understood as to understand,
To be loved as to love.
For it is in giving that we receive,
It is in pardoning that we are pardoned,
And it is in dying that we are born to eternal life.

FACT

Every spiritual tradition places peace at the center of its practical life. Peace with oneself is extended to one's fellows. This, in turn, is believed to influence society at large, and the world as a whole. In Muslim cultures, people greet each other with *Salaam*; in Jewish communities, *Shalom*; in Hindu countries, *Namaste*; in Polynesia, *Aloha*. These words share the same meaning, "Peace be unto you."

The Spiritual Betrothal of Teresa of Ávila

By the sixteenth century, monastic life for women was widespread in Europe. Influential intellects and mystics moved toward the contemplative life, away from the continually changing fortunes of political institutions throughout the region. Among them was a young Spanish woman, Teresa de Cepeda y Ahumada, born in 1515.

Although she became known for her reforms of the Carmelite order, St. Teresa's spiritual enlightenment emphasized a new concept: orison, the practice of silent prayer. She viewed this as an act of worship itself and an expression of love. Through this, the individual maintains the "spiritual betrothal" that exists between the soul and God: "We might say that this is as if the ends of two wax candles were joined so that the light they give us is one . . . or it is as if a tiny streamlet enters the sea, from which it will find no way of separating itself . . ."

St. Teresa passed away in 1582. Her works, *The Way of Perfection* and *The Interior Castle*, recount her teachings on mystical prayer to the sisters of her order. In 1970, she became the first woman to be named Doctor of the Church.

The Jesus Prayer and Hesychasm

Nikodimos Hagioritis (1748–1809) was a Greek orthodox monk who brought about a spiritual renaissance through his writings on "the love of the good and beautiful." He entered on this devotional path initially to translate the writings of the Eastern Orthodox church; but on spiritual pilgrimages through Greece and Turkey, he discovered the "prayer of the heart." This is perpetual prayer, the continual recitation of the name of Jesus. By performing this prayer constantly, Nikodimos taught that the mind would relinquish its attachment to the world and come to rest in the heart. Here, it is possible to enter the divine state.

FACT

One of the meanings of grace is: "an excellence or a power granted by God." However, some Christian mystics believe that grace always exists and merely becomes accessible through prayer. If we are not innately good, then we must look outside ourselves for grace. If we are innately good, then we must learn how to unlock the grace that is within.

This revelation is recorded in his prodigious work, the *Philokalia*. It was to later influence an anonymous Russian writer in the mid-nineteenth century who produced the classical spiritual novel, *The Way of a Pilgrim*. It recounts the journey of a seeker who attains spiritual realization by reciting the prayer, "Lord Jesus Christ, Son of God, have pity on me."

The Starsi

The approach to prayer that Nikodimos Hagioritis taught was actually a revival of mystical tradition practiced by the Starsi, who came from middle Russia. Though initially a monastic teaching, it was also offered to laypersons who lived in close proximity to the Starsi.

Here, prayers and divine names are repeated in order to purify oneself of images and distracting thoughts. It is essentially the practice of *hesychia*, a way of emptying the mundane self and filling it with divine presence at the same time.

This form of prayer follows the model of Christ in the Phillipians hymn (Chapter 2.6–7 NRSV), which says of Jesus:

> *Though he was in the form of God,*
> *did not regard equality with God as something to be exploited,*
> *but emptied himself,*
> *taking the form of a slave,*
> *being born in human likeness.*

The hesychast empties herself of all thoughts and concepts in order to be filled with the divine, in imitation of the suffering Christ. The method of the Jesus prayer works by subtracting all that does not conform to the ideal of regenerated humanity represented by Christ. The term for this regeneration in the Orthodox church is *theosis*, or divinization, the freely given, abundant gift of sharing life with God before the death of the body. Theosis is often compared to polishing a tarnished mirror: the image of God is always there underneath—it just needs to be revealed through spiritual cultivation.

Thomas Merton and the Twentieth Century

In recent times, a renaissance of contemplative prayer emerged from the inspirational poetry and art of the Trappist monk Father Lewis, known to the public as Thomas Merton. Born in 1915, Merton came to the United States from France in the 1930s to study and teach. Although he had been agnostic in early life, he converted to Catholicism and left the teaching profession for a life of solitude as a monk. He chose the Trappists, the popular name for a branch of the Cistercian order founded in seventeenth-century France. Their rule is very strict—seclusion, minimal food, meatless diet, hard labor, and a vow of silence. However, this has not prevented their members from pursuing artistic and social endeavors. In that spirit, Merton produced best-selling social commentaries and religious works in the form of prayers, poetry, and meditations.

QUOTE

"Let there always be quiet, dark churches in which people can take refuge . . . houses of God filled with his silent presence. There, even when they do not know how to pray, at least they can be still and breathe easily."

—Thomas Merton

The Abbey of Our Lady of Gethsemane near Bardstown, Kentucky, became Merton's home, where he taught students and novices. He wrote about learning stillness through "centering prayer," and about a concept shared by many meditative paths, the "final integration." Merton believed that final integration brings every person in contact with his or her true nature, a divine nature.

Merton became a close friend of Thich Nhat Hanh, the Vietnamese Zen Buddhist monk who proposed the idea of engaged (socially active) Buddhism. Merton passed away in 1968 in Bangkok, Thailand, while attending an ecumenical conference of Buddhist and Christian monks. Today, Thomas Merton contemplative retreats are offered around the world and a foundation disseminates his works and teachings. On his experience in prayer, Merton wrote, "Contemplation is the perfection of love and knowledge."

Sacred Heart Meditation and Adoration of the Host

Devotion to the Sacred Heart of Jesus began with Saint Mary Margaret Alcoque (1647–1690), a nun of the Visitation Order. According to Margaret

Mary, Jesus appeared to her and offered his heart as a refuge for human-kind, promising her that whoever kept an image of the heart visible in the home would be granted fulfillment of several promises. Among these promises were the fulfillment of material needs fitting to the person's station in life, peace in family matters, speed in the perfection of sanctity, and consolation in life and death. The forms of the devotion came to vary greatly over the centuries, but they often include a litany like the following:

Heart of Jesus, of infinite majesty, have mercy on us.
Heart of Jesus, holy temple of God, have mercy on us,
Heart of Jesus, house of God and gate of Heaven, have mercy on us,
Heart of Jesus, glowing furnace of charity, have mercy on us,
Heart of Jesus, full of goodness and love, have mercy on us,
Heart of Jesus, abyss of all virtues, have mercy on us.

A closely related practice is the veneration of the host, the sanctified bread and wine kept in the sanctuary. Because these, too, are held to partake in the life of Christ, they are venerated with silent and verbal prayers.

The Mysteries of the Rosary

One of the most important Catholic devotions, increasingly practiced by other Christians as well, is the Holy Rosary. The rosary can be a fruitful way of prayer or meditation when you don't know what words to say or when meditating in silence becomes too difficult. The rosary can also be a big help when you feel "stuck" in some particular life situation or spiritual problem.

The rosary can be said in twenty or thirty minutes, or it can take hours. It all depends on the amount of time spent ruminating on each prayer. The scenes from scripture can actually be read or simply recalled on the indicated beads. As for the rosary itself, you can buy a set of plastic beads for a few dollars or an ornate strand for hundreds of dollars. Try to purchase one that will not be so fragile that it breaks after one or two uses and can stand up to being placed in a pocket. Traditionally, a rosary should be blessed by a priest and should not be worn as jewelry. It can be said before a candle or an image of Jesus, Mary, or a favorite saint.

There are several prayers that are repeated as the Rosary is said:

The Apostles' Creed

I believe in God, the Father Almighty, maker of Heaven and Earth, and in Jesus Christ, his Son, Our Lord. He was born of the Virgin Mary, suffered under Pontius Pilate, was crucified, dead, and buried. He descended into Hell. On the third day he arose again, ascended into Heaven, and sits at the right hand of God the Father Almighty. From thence he shall come to judge the living and the dead. I believe in the Holy Catholic Church, the communion of saints, the forgiveness of sins, the resurrection of the body, and the life everlasting. Amen.

The Glory Be (Gloria Patri)

Glory be to the Father, and to the Son, and to the Holy Spirit. As it was in the beginning, is now, and ever shall be. World without end. Amen.

Hail Mary

Hail Mary, full of grace, the Lord is with thee. Blessed art thou among women, and blessed is the fruit of thy womb, Jesus. Holy Mary, Mother of God, pray for us sinners, both now and at the hour of our death. Amen.

Our Father (The Lord's Prayer)

Our Father, who art in Heaven, hallowed be thy name. Thy kingdom come, thy will be done, on Earth as it is in Heaven. Give us this day our daily bread, and forgive us our trespasses, as we forgive those who trespass against us, and lead us not into temptation, but deliver us from evil (for thine is the kingdom, and the power, and the glory forever). Amen.

Hail Holy Queen

Hail holy Queen, mother of mercy, our life, our sweetness, and our hope. To thee do we cry, poor banished children of Eve. To thee do we send up our sighs, moaning, and weeping in this vale of tears. Turn then, most gracious Advocate, your eyes of mercy toward us. Show to us the blessed fruit of your womb, Jesus. Oh, clement, oh loving, oh sweet Virgin Mary. Amen.

Oh, My Jesus

Oh, My Jesus, forgive us our sins and lead all souls into Heaven, especially those most in need of your mercy. Amen.

▼ **MYSTERIES OF THE HOLY ROSARY**

Joyful Mysteries	Sorrowful Mysteries	Glorious Mysteries	Luminous Mysteries
Monday and Saturday	Tuesday and Friday	Wednesday and Sunday	Thursday
1.The Annunciation	1. The Agony in the Garden	1. The Resurrection	1. The Baptism in the Jordan
2. The Visitation	2. The Scourging at the Pillar	2. The Ascension	2. The Wedding At Cana
3. The Birth of Jesus	3. The Crowning with Thorns	3. Coming of the Holy Ghost	3. The Proclamation of the Kingdom
4. The Presentation of Jesus in the Temple	4. The Carrying of the Cross	4. The Assumption of Mary into Heaven	4. The Transfiguration
5. The Finding of Jesus in the Temple	5. Crucifixion and Death of Jesus	5. The Crowning of Mary	5. The Institution of the Eucharist
Scripture: John 2	Luke 1–2	Matthew 26–27	John 20; Luke 24; Acts 2 Matthew 3, 17, 26

HOW TO SAY THE ROSARY:

1. On the cross or crucifix, say the Apostles' Creed.
2. On the first bead, say one Lord's Prayer.
3. Say Hail Mary three times.
4. On the last invitatory bead, say the Glory Be and announce the first Mystery (Example: "The First Mystery is The Baptism in the Jordan"). Then say The Lord's Prayer.
5. Say Hail Mary ten times while meditating on the first Mystery.
6. On the next set, say the Glory Be, announce the second Mystery, and say The Lord's Prayer.
7. Say Ten Hail Marys. Repeat the process for the third, fourth, and fifth Mysteries.
8. To conclude, say the Glory Be, Oh My Jesus, and Hail Holy Queen.

The rosary is a meditative tour through the gospel story as viewed through the eyes of Mary. Most people probably think of the rosary as a Roman Catholic devotion, and that is its largest audience. But the words of the prayers themselves and the gospel events in the Mysteries are derived from scripture and are important for all Christians. Those outside the Christian tradition may also find the prayers meaningful, since Christ was, after all, a human being. His life and sufferings have something to do with all of us. If anyone can practice Zen meditation, why can't anyone say the rosary?

Walking the Labyrinth

The labyrinth is a medieval devotion that has been revived in recent decades. An intricate geometrical pattern originally built into the floor of a cathedral, the labyrinth allows the faithful to make metaphorical pilgrimage to Jerusalem without leaving home. The center of the circular pattern represents Jerusalem, and the seeker must reach the center by means of the circuitous outside pathways. The labyrinth is not a maze: the path will lead to the center if followed long enough, and there are no dead ends or detours. Psychologically, though, the labyrinth plays on the walker's expectations, as the way that seems to be close to the center will often lead right back to the outer edge again.

If walked with intention, the labyrinth becomes a way of bodily prayer. It can become a complex form of introspection, or it can simply be a few minutes spent in silence. Students of religion will find the comparisons to yogic yantras and Tibetan mandalas to be striking. Churches in major metropolitan areas will often have a labyrinth available for walking, and portable versions, printed on canvas, are also available. Walking the labyrinth can be a good way to mark the beginning or end of a retreat, prepare for a worship service or meditation group, or get rid of nagging distractions and doubts. This deceptively simple, traditional devotion will allow you to walk your way to your own center as you walk through the labyrinth.

The Language of Christian Mysticism

As you study Christian mysticism, you're likely to come across the following terms:

- **Anchorite:** One who lives a contemplative life in solitude
- **Apocrypha:** Books that have not been included in the Old and New Testaments because of their lack of authentication
- **Charismatic:** Someone who believes he has been visited by the Holy Spirit as the apostles were at the Pentecost
- **Heresy:** Religious beliefs that are not compatible with the authorized teachings of the Church
- **Monophysite:** A belief, maintained by the Eastern (Orthodox) church but rejected by the Western (Catholic) church in the sixth century, that Christ's human and divine natures were not separate, but one

CHAPTER 15

A Feast for the Eyes

Visual images are very important, because the mind is attentive in the here and now. So anything that presents itself while in this state will reflect in the mind quite readily. Artists through the ages have also recognized this and presented us with their inspirations, fears, and acerbic depictions of human life to provoke our thinking.

A Picture Is Worth a Thousand Petals

The mind has other powers besides perceiving and analyzing. Imagination drives many human endeavors; without it, there would be no progress. Science, art, and religion would not exist, because the creative mind produces concepts and activities that allow us to explore all the dimensions of life that lie above and below our consciousness.

Imagery can similarly power the experience of stillness. All of the meditation traditions have an established branch that uses pictures, designs, and icons to convey certain goals for the practitioner. While they are regarded only as temporary devices, images are important for a number of reasons:

- **Centering:** Images focus attention on one idea.
- **Contemplation:** Illustrations may reflect a particular quality that the meditator seeks.
- **Guidance:** Diagrams act as "spiritual maps," depicting the topography of the mind, the soul, or the universe.
- **Integration:** Designs draw attention to the interrelationship of ideas.
- **Inspiration:** Pictures inspire exalted states of mind or feeling.

Meditation and Imagery

Yogic and Buddhist meditation environments make great use of imagery to fulfill some of the goals sought by the practitioner. One visual aid is the *yantra* ("support"), a linear diagram that supports a visualization. It is usually geometric and symmetrical, combining circles with squares and joining the lines inside and outside each figure. This design conveys the idea of order, harmony, and balance. The *yantra* is used for centering, and in Tantric practice it is believed to offer protection. The meditator places her conscious presence in the center, where it is "shielded" from interferences of thought and feeling.

Yantras are drawn on walls, curtains, and tablets that are placed in the meditation environment. A limited number of colors are used; each color symbolizes a particular state of mind and cosmic activity.

The mandala ("circle") is also a diagram that can feature images of deities, plants, and animals. Each image has a symbolic meaning that imparts qualities of mind to the meditator. The mandala conveys synthesis and integration, showing how relationships exist between the meditator and the elements in the image. Concentric circles are used to depict levels or layers of reality, symbolizing the meditator's journey into the inner realms. In this respect, the mandala is also a map of those regions.

In the Buddhist tradition, mandalas are viewed as magical objects. The meditator, if practiced enough, may "absorb" the qualities of the image and through the process, receive healing or special illuminations.

Buddhism emphasizes the "middle way" of the Buddha. He learned that the extremes in life are dead ends and only perpetuate themselves. Wealth and poverty, indulgence and austerity, are two sides of one coin. Instead, he taught that attaining enlightenment is important, but applying it to the world of reality is equally significant. This is the middle way.

Mandalas are sometimes three-dimensional. In the Tibetan tradition, these images are created from dyed sand and plant materials such as rice and seeds. They are carefully arranged in intricate designs on floors, tables, and cushions for special ceremonies. When the event is over, the materials are gathered and returned to nature.

Religious images are important imagery devices in meditation. Statues or pictures of saints, angels, bodhisattvas, and deities inspire depressed or painful states of mind. Through contemplation, they also illuminate solutions for the meditator. Buddhist *thangkas* and icons of the Orthodox Christian Church are images that represent powers or graces for particular circumstances or conditions.

A Visual Meditation

Whichever form of imagery you choose for meditation, you may follow a simple, fifteen-minute process for allowing it to assist in the goals you are pursuing.

View the image overall for about five minutes, allowing it to "impress" on you. Do not seek detail; see it as a whole. Close your eyes and see the overall image in your mind. If you can't "see" it with your eyes closed, open your eyes and return to the image once more. For the next five minutes, allow your attention to seek the details of the image. A constructive approach is to begin at the base (six o'clock position) and continue in a clockwise direction. You may notice colors, designs, numbers of petals on the flowers, and symbols within the image. Close your eyes and see the details in your mind, repeating the clockwise motion. Continue this process for the second five minutes or until the image is firmly established in your mind. In the last five minutes, sit quietly, waiting for any message that the image might have for you.

Images in the Mystical Jewish Tradition

Judaism arose more than 4,000 years ago in what is now the State of Israel as a divine covenant between God and the ancient Hebrews. Two important books provide the dogma of Judaism. The Torah (also called the Pentateuch) is based on the first five books of the Old Testament and teaches the law of the Hebrew religion. The Talmud is a collection of commentaries on the Torah, interpreting the law.

Like every religion, Judaism is mostly known by its orthodox dogma and practices, but it also has an esoteric dimension. It is outlined in the Kabbalah ("tradition"), the third book of Judaism that provides the contemplative vehicle of the tradition. It is a body of knowledge that discloses the structure of the universe and its relation to human consciousness.

The Kabbalah itself consists primarily of two texts that reveal the esoteric tradition of Israel. They are the *Sepher Yetzirah* ("*Book of Formation*") and the *Sepher ha Zohar* ("*Book of Splendor*"). They date from the second century and were carried to Europe in the Middle Ages where medieval philosophers added appendices with numerous commentaries. These were revived in the early twentieth century by metaphysical movements in Europe, particularly the Order of the Golden Dawn and in America, by the Theosophists.

The essence of kabbalistic teaching is the *Otz Chiim* ("tree of life"). It is a sort of master plan of the universe, but it is also a map through the inner worlds that guides the mystic traveler. The Tree of Life is a meditative image, a mandala of the universe and the soul in one symbol. Recalling the narrative in Genesis of the Tree of Good and Evil, the story may be viewed as an allegory of the separation of the spirit and matter when physical life came into being.

The reunion of those two worlds is the goal of the meditator in this system. It is accomplished by following the "paths" that are outlined in the Tree of Life.

There are ten individual *sephira* ("worlds") that compose the Tree of Life. They are arranged in three vertical rows or "pillars," representing the three modes of approach. Those modes are active, passive, and modulating. The meditator is guided as much as possible upward, through the middle path or pillar. This approach avoids extremes of mental and emotional experience.

Going up through the worlds in the "Tree of the Sephiroth," the meditator also moves through four levels or planes of cosmic activity: *Assiah, Yetzirah, Briah,* and *Aziluth.* These are, progressing upward, the states of physical life, angelic life (nature spirits included), the created universe (celestial bodies and forces), and the region of divine beings, respectively. They also symbolize layers of consciousness, which could be compared to the four states of consciousness in Yoga (deep sleep, dreaming, waking consciousness, and divine consciousness). Let's look at the individual worlds of the Sephirothic Tree to understand this view of the meditative path.

- We begin in the state of *Assiah* ("physical life") and first encounter *Malkuth* ("the kingdom"), the entry gate on the path to illumination. In this world there are the four elements. Their colors are citrine, brown, and gray. This is where the body exists and the natural world finds expression.
- From *Assiah,* we enter the state of *Yetzirah* ("immaterial life"). In *Yesod* ("the foundation"), we encounter the tidal ebb and flow, the region of shadowy images that mirror life in the material world. The color is purple. *Hod* ("splendor") is where we discover luminous perception, a clarity of thought and the senses. The color is orange. In *Netzach* ("victory"), the world of harmony and achievement is experienced. The color is green.
- From *Yetzirah,* we enter the state of *Briah* ("the cosmic world"). *Tipareth* ("beauty") is the central Sun, the illumination of nature's source. The color is yellow. *Geburah* ("severity") is the solar system, a tightly wound mechanism of matter and energy in motion. The color is red. *Chesed* ("mercy") is the galaxies, ever-expanding clusters of stars that are born and die in eons of time. The color is blue.

- From *Briah,* we come into the state of *Aziluth* ("divine consciousness"). *Binah* ("understanding") is the cosmic mother, where creation is brought forth. The color is violet. *Chokmah* ("wisdom") is the cosmic father, where the impulse of life emanates. The color is indigo. *Kether* ("the crown") is the source of all creation, the matrix of spirit. The color is white.

Beyond *Kether* lies the *Ain Soph Aur,* the "limitless light." It is the primeval beginning of the universe, the unknowable.

QUOTE

"All that is seen—heaven, earth, and all that fills it—all these things are the external garments of God."
—Shneur Zalman of Liadi (1745–1813), one of the founders of the Hasidic movement

Color Meditation

The power of all imagery depends to a great extent on the impact of the colors that constitute the picture. Psychologists, design experts, and healers all agree that the colors around us deeply affect our perceptions. They convey states of mind that are initially perceived visually but gradually filter into our thinking and feeling. A number of approaches to working with color have developed in modern times. Colors have been used in factories to enhance the productivity of workers. Colors are also used to reduce aggression or depression in institutions. Chromatherapy, or color healing, is used to influence the balance of the body when illness affects functioning and recovery. Many of the current systems were derived from the study of the ancient meditation traditions and how color is used in those systems to harmonize the mind.

Utilizing Color in Meditation

Colors may be visualized in meditation for healing and maintaining certain states of mind. First, create a "color zone" where you can initially focus on color themes. It should face a blank wall or curtain of a neutral shade, so that there is no other visual interference. Buy a sturdy easel that can be placed at eye level in your meditation oasis. For this, select colors of matte board that can be cut into medium-size pieces, either 8" × 10" or 9" × 12". Many suppliers have odd cuts for sale, so there is no need to buy a full sheet.

Place the board on the easel in your meditation oasis. It should be to the right or left of your sitting area, but not in front of it. You want to be able to move your attention elsewhere if necessary.

In chromatherapy, lamps are used to fill a small area with colored light. The person may sit or sleep in the area, and in some instances the lamp is focused directly on an affected part of the body. This is a different practice from visualization, in which the mind is trained to evoke color and recall it during meditation. The two are not the same practice.

Devote at least fifteen minutes to a color session. As with the imagery meditation, give the overall subject a distant gaze for the first five minutes, then close your eyes. Look at the subject with attention to detail for the next five minutes, and then close your eyes. Gaze at the overall subject again for the last five minutes.

Choosing Colors

Color meditation should be limited to one color per session to allow the color to affect mental and emotional levels.

Red is associated with fire, blood, and vitality. It is the most stimulating of the colors and should be used sparingly in the meditation environment. However, red is also required for clarity of mind when problem solving and raising physical strength after an illness. It stimulates the immune functions and should be followed shortly afterward with a green or blue visualization.

Orange is associated with action, excitement, and warmth. Combining the life force of red with the liveliness of yellow, orange imparts a sense of well-being and regeneration. It is said to influence the body's organs to function optimally, and is especially good for digestion. Use orange as a rising agent for emotions and as a mental restorative.

The breath of life is seen in yellow by many cultures. It has a positive effect on the nervous system and stimulates thinking and communication. It is a natural antidepressant, as researchers who study seasonal affective disorder (SAD) have discovered.

Green is the color of nature, growth, and balance. It is a natural tonic while it invites relaxation. The body's rhythms are calmed by green. Use it for "grounding" yourself to the present circumstances. Green also assists in emotional poise and balance.

Blue has a cooling effect and counters excited or fearful states of mind. Blue is the color of peace and reflection. Use blue for tranquility, especially after a lot of mental activity. It also instills aspiration and dignity.

FACT

In some tarot teachings, the student is advised to paint or color a complete set of seventy-eight images for meditative use. Black-and-white decks are available for this purpose, along with instruction guides on the coloring procedure. In essence, the work is a process of visually "giving life" to the images inscribed on the cards by simultaneously infusing color and focusing attention.

Violet combines vitality (red) and serenity (blue). Violet is the color of spirituality. Use it sparingly, however, because it can promote an "otherworldliness" that is not practical. Idealism and intuitive powers are associated with violet.

Combining Color and Breath for Health

Following the visualization of color, the experienced meditator may employ a set of *pranayama* breathing exercises. This technique is used therapeutically to remedy chronic health problems.

Start by performing the color visualization exercise. Then begin the color breathing exercise. Take slow, moderately deep breaths. Allow yourself five minutes to do this. As you inhale, visualize the color on the easel lifting off and entering the body, circulating through it. As you exhale, the color fills the space around you and becomes part of the body aura. This may be done to "carry" the color's influence for a time.

Mystical Meditation with the Tarot

The tarot is one of the mystical tools that convey powerful images for meditation. It is thought to be a codex of the kabbalistic Tree of Life, and there are many sources that show the relationship between the seventy-eight images and the Sephiroth. There is evidence, although obscure, that the system was used for divination in the Middle Ages. Occult legend has it that around 200 B.C.E., the sages of Alexandria, Egypt, recognized the ending of the pagan age. So they fabricated the system to preserve the wisdom of the ancients in visual form. By placing the system in a deck of playing cards, the sages knew the knowledge could never be lost because the human proclivity for gambling would never cease.

ESSENTIAL

As you meditate on each image, observe the gestures of the figures, the colors, and the numerical symbolism. You may also use the images to evoke certain states of mind.

Tarot images can awaken the senses and imagination. Every image in the seventy-eight-card deck has symbolic meaning. Besides the representations of divine beings, humans engaged in everyday tasks, and animals, there are numbers, colors, and names that have esoteric significance. The knowledge encrypted in the cards is so vast that only meditation can truly unlock it. Experienced tarot masters say that after years of working with these images, new insights continue to present themselves.

The cards in the tarot are divided into two realms: the minor arcana and the major arcana. The minor arcana reflect the arrangement of suits in traditional playing cards: wands (clubs), swords (spades), cups (hearts), and pentacles (diamonds), each with ten numbered and four court cards. These cards convey the images of transitory conditions. The major arcana (sometimes referred to as the "trumps") are distinctive. Numbered from zero to twenty-one (twenty-two in all), they convey images of universal conditions.

Why twenty-two figures? Recalling the kabbalistic Tree of the Sephiroth, there are ten worlds or spheres that represent universal conditions. Joining these ten spheres are the "paths" that lead to their knowledge. There are twenty-two paths in all, and they are symbolized by the major arcana in the tarot. When viewed in sequence, the paths lead "up the tree" of knowledge of good and evil.

Among other things, each of the major arcana cards represents the path to using the cosmic powers for personal growth. In this sense, they are excellent keys to use in seed meditation. The cards are also believed to convey wisdom subconsciously, which will lead to more acute "readings" when they are consulted for divinatory answers in nonmeditation settings.

Meditating with Tarot Cards

Approach meditation with tarot images in sequence. Begin with 0 (The Fool); end with 21 (The World). The sequence is important, because it represents the progression of cosmic wisdom from the general to the particular spheres of your experience. Even the cards that don't seem pleasing should be included in their natural sequence.

You may begin the sequence with one image for a very short period in one meditation session and go on to the next until you have finished with all twenty-two. Alternately, you may use one for each day of meditation sequentially, or even one image for a month of meditation sessions. No matter how much time you allow for each image, you can always return to the beginning and start the sequence again. You can learn a lot each time you use the tarot; for some, it is a continuous exercise in symbolic thinking.

Understanding the Powers in the Tarot Images

Each of the tarot images provides information or "lessons" of personal power. They are conveyed through the colors, figures, and actions depicted in the scenes on each card.

0: The Fool—Fortitude, Enthusiasm. *Your insight is awakened into new situations and unfamiliar conditions. In spite of this, your sense of humor and spontaneity come forward, reminding you that you are free to use your will imaginatively.*

1: The Magician—Coordination, Synchronization. *The order you seek in your life arrives, as well as the skill to translate raw materials into* objects of usefulness and beauty. You are in control of your realm, yet still adaptable to new ways of thinking.

2: The High Priestess—Intuition, Retention. *You are presented with the scroll of the Akashic record, the cosmic memory of all things past, present, and future. You are able to fuse objectivity with feeling, so that you may use this power to make wise decisions and guide others.*

3: The Empress—Empathy, Affection. *You enter the realm of the Divine Mother, who impels all around her to flourish. She celebrates and shares the fruits of her creative garden with you. You become warm and resourceful, bringing a continuous expression of beauty, harmony, and passion in your labors.*

4: The Emperor—Organization, Leadership. *You become strongly connected to your instincts, and keen on assessing people and ideas. You are resistant to harmful influences in thought, health, and your environment.*

5: The Hierophant—Cultivation, Enhancement. *Like the ancient priest, you draw people together in harmony and peace. You encourage their endeavors, and convey wisdom whenever you teach or speak. There are wondrous products of art, architecture, and tradition wherever you are found.*

6: The Lovers—Harmony, Loyalty. *An angelic spirit overshadows your relationships, blessing the efforts you make with others. You are able to see through the petty concerns of daily life and see the big picture that you are both working toward.*

7: The Chariot—Advancement, Initiative. *You are able to maintain a forward movement that brings change and adaptation in your life. You are unmoving in your resolve, even though everything around you is in motion. Your resolve also gives you the empathy to understand and guide others forward.*

8: Strength—Control, Persistence. *The exalted being who restrains the lion is the power you possess to overcome all difficulties. Your commitment to staying on the path you have chosen will be fulfilled in the most auspicious manner.*

9: The Hermit—Restraint, Discipline. *Circumspection will bring insight into your life, so that you may reflect on meanings and truths. Through your endeavors you will be patient, and reminded that everything will take place in its proper time for the best results.*

10: The Wheel of Fortune—Adaptability, Versatility. *You will approach your challenges with imagination and optimism. Nothing in your life will stay the same; change will allow you to use your talents and receive rewards for your resourcefulness.*

11: Justice—Objectivity, Equanimity. *There will be balance between your thoughts and actions, and your objectivity will prevail. You will exercise fairness in your dealings, although you must be detached from the confused thoughts and feelings of others.*

12: The Hanged Man—Compassion, Idealism. *All that has worried you can be seen as transitory and insignificant compared to your vast inner resources. That which you have placed highest in your life will be achieved in time.*

13: Death—Insight, Sensitivity. *You will discover that your fears are groundless, and that sunrise always follows a dark night. Conditions that appear distressing are transformed into opportunities for valuable experience.*

14: Temperance—Moderating, Discriminating. *Your angelic presence encourages you to weigh all factors when making choices. You must balance the material and spiritual goals in your life so that you may enjoy progress in both realms.*

15: The Devil—Tenacity, Dynamism. *Although there is a price to pay for every material possession, your dynamic force can be directed to the work that calls for it. You will make the proper choices in this realm and not be fettered by regret.*

16: The Tower—Swift Action, Dedication. *Clarity of mind will allow you to maintain calm amidst the storm. Falsehoods will become obvious, and truth will guide you to courageous action for resolving complex problems.*

17: The Star—Optimism, Tolerance. *Despite setbacks, your hopes will arrive at a favorable destination. Sharing your insights with others, you overcome misunderstandings that have blocked your inner vision.*

18: The Moon—Detachment, Impersonality. *In a world of confusion, you exercise clarity. This draws others who wish to flee from their problems to you, but you gently guide them toward resolutions.*

19: The Sun—Generosity, Humor, Devotion. *A return to the carefree world of youth and vitality is possible. By accepting yourself with all strengths and weaknesses, you are renewed in spirit.*

20: Judgment—Dedication, Resolution. *No matter what obstacles you face, the inner strength to overcome them is accessible to you. Your goals are meaningful and important.*

21: The World—Patience, Endurance. *Your life exists in harmonious balance, irrespective of change and appearances. Within this harmony, you realize the illusion of time and understand eternal values.*

Creative Visualization

There are a number of approaches to meditation that use "creative visualization." This method focuses on images that arise from your own imagination, not an external source (images, sounds, sensations). For example, a meditation exercise may begin with the suggestion to visualize a stream of water slowly coursing down a mountain.

As simple as this suggestion sounds, many are not able to visualize it. This is because some people are more verbal than visual, or more apt to hear unrecorded music in the mind than conjure abstract pictures. Everyone's creative sense is "bent" in one or more directions; few people use it the same way. This is normal, and nothing to worry about.

Learning how to use creative visualization can assist in a wider meditation practice, and it's worth devoting some time to mastering it. Creative visualization takes place with closed eyes. The first step is to immediately place yourself in the picture, before anything else. For example, when you are given the cue to be on a mountain, first see yourself on the mountain.

Still in the picture, gradually look outside yourself. Look out of your eyes in this scene, seeing your hands and feet, all of your body, the clothing you are wearing. Now look at the vista. See yourself on the mountain, looking down at the view. Looking up, see the sky. Looking around you, see the brush, trees, and rocks. Maintain your presence on the mountain for as long as possible, at least ten minutes. Coming back to the present, perform the visualization in reverse. Seeing the landscape, look up at the sky; then look down at your clothing, body, hands, and feet. Then open your eyes.

ESSENTIAL

Establish a consistent meditation practice to get the most out of creative visualization. Then, use creative visualization sessions periodically to set the goals you establish into motion. The Idea here is not to impose new challenges every time you meditate.

Creative visualization is best done on your own, following a script that you may compose and then read or tape for playback in a meditation session. Many of the commercially prerecorded scripts do now allow enough time for the imaginative faculty of the meditator to engage in constructing and maintaining the picture. Tracks number 1, 3, and 4 on the CD that accompanies this book will involve elements of creative visualization.

It is also important to reverse the visualization after you've gone through it, before you open your eyes and return to ordinary activity. Otherwise, if the visualization is particularly foreign (like imagining a dragon in flight), you may feel disoriented. Think of it as taking a journey. You go along a new path, but you want to return to your starting place.

Creative visualization is useful for guiding your attention to specific goals. It plays an important part in healing, learning, and relaxation, but it does not use the full scope of awareness that meditation uses.

CHAPTER 16

Music, Mantra, and Meditation

Sound lies at the very root of human communication, and has before the written word ever came into being. Sounds viscerally impact our bodies: we can't help moving to the rhythms that we hear. Spiritual traditions harness the power of sound to bring subtle changes in consciousness that would otherwise be unavailable.

Sound and Creation

Clearing the mind is the initial challenge of meditation. To address this, repetitive sounds and words have been used in meditative and mystical practices through the ages. They are believed to aid in spiritual focus, as a means of maintaining a particular frame of mind or feeling. Words and sounds are also equated with metaphorical actions. For example, "Abracadabra" is a legendary magical word that is reputed to change lead into gold. It is the same for "Open Sesame," the magical phrase that revealed the cave of the robber chief in *Ali Baba and the Forty Thieves*. Such words are metaphors for opening the mind to the hidden treasures within.

QUOTE

"Happiness is not a matter of intensity but of balance and order and rhythm and harmony."

—Thomas Merton

Nearly all traditions cite the creation of the world as an act of sound or exhalation of breath. The Latin *spiritus* and the Greek *pneuma* indicate both breath and spirit. The Hindus envision the god Shiva emoting *spanda,* the cosmic rhythm of the universe, as he dances an eternal dance of life. The ancient Egyptians believed that when the god Thoth spoke the word of creation, all things vibrated into being. In Genesis, creation is brought into being at God's utterance. In all these cosmogonies, the world manifests through sound or vibration, continuing to expand in the resonance produced by the initial creative utterance.

Modern science is looking at the effect of sound in new ways. Laboratory studies show that music and rhythm can affect cellular life in positive or negative ways depending on the sounds. In therapeutic settings and learning environments, we are beginning to see how important sound is for clearing the mind and preparing it to receive new information. The meditator can also use sound to initiate a resonance that sets the stage for a positive meditative experience. There are as many approaches to using sound as there are meditative styles. You can create your own sound program by listening to what is traditionally used and incorporating what "sounds right" to you.

Perhaps you feel drawn to a particular hymn or bhajan, perhaps an opera aria or a samba beat interests you, or maybe you feel more at ease with the blues or spirituals.

The Rhythm of the Brain

Sound and rhythm are wired into the human body. Electrical impulses between nerve cells produce all activity in the brain, the control center of the body. These impulses are measured in hertz, or cycles per second. In modern times, researchers have correlated specific states of consciousness with the number of cycles produced by brain waves. Brain waves are grouped into four categories: delta, theta, alpha, and beta. However, current research is refining these categories as scientists learn more about the mind, the body, and consciousness.

Delta State: The delta state, which consists of waves of 0.5 to 4.0 cycles per second, is found in deep sleep. This is the lowest cycle observed. In this state, the mind is not attentive to anything in the outside world.

Theta State: The theta state, which consists of waves of 4 to 8 cycles per second, is found in light sleep and deep meditation. This is a "bridge state" between tranquility and drifting off into unconsciousness. Daydreams occur here, as well as events in which the person is conscious but unable to recall details.

Alpha State: The alpha state, in which the waves are 8 to 12 cycles per second, is a relaxed state of nonarousal. Thinking disturbs the alpha state, but attention is active. Reflection and contemplation are associated with this category; it is the target state in most meditation and biofeedback exercises. The normal resting heart rate is about 72 beats per minute. The same rhythm is believed to induce a state of relaxation in alpha state, and if emulated in music, it can be very hypnotic.

Beta State: The beta state, consisting of waves of 12 to 16 cycles per second, is associated with the engaged mind. Speaking, relating to others, learning a new skill—these activities fall into the beta state.

Meditation moves the mind away from the highly active wavelengths and into the contemplative and reflective wavelengths. Just imagine trying to relax when a road crew is operating a jackhammer outside your window. In the same way, the meditative frame of mind is best reached when the external sounds are conducive to this state and the internal wavelengths in the brain are cooperating. Music and mantra can help facilitate the transition to the deeper, more reflective states.

FACT

High beta, with waves of 16 to 32 cycles per second, denotes high emotion such as fear or excitement. The mind is focused on specifics, situations that may be either desirable or threatening. The super-high beta state, with waves of 35 to 150 cycles per second, was only recently discovered.

Mantra: The Sacred Formula

Sound is an integral part of meditative work in many traditions, and for some it is sacred language. Sound is a mystical science in Yoga and a focusing device in all branches of Buddhism. In these practices, certain tones, spoken or intoned, assist in narrowing attention. In Sufism, Judaism, and Christianity, these tones take the form of recitation of sacred names and phrases to achieve a centered state and oneness with the spirit. Chant is also an important part of both religious and secular life in all of the indigenous religions of Africa, Asia, the South Pacific, and the Americas. It unifies the mind of a tribe, while preserving some of the culture's history and beliefs.

Sound and music evoke certain states of mind that reflect mythological and universal themes. Here are some examples:

- **The Creator:** Sounds that evoke the creative nature, placing the person at the center of the environment; chants, invocations, and holy names fortify the will and self-awareness.
- **The Peacemaker:** Sounds that promote harmony and tranquility, allowing everyone to meet in agreement; hymns and ballads are often expressions of peace.
- **The Unifier:** Sounds that join people together in the same spirit of thinking or feeling; prayers and songs that proclaim divine qualities

unify people; words of inspiration and courage like national anthems and military marches also fall into this category.

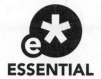

ESSENTIAL

Om is a Sanskrit word with many meanings, though it embodies the life force in all its manifestations. Although it is spelled *o-m*, it is vocalized differently, in three syllables *a-u-m*, and pronounced Aauu-ooo-mm. These three syllables represent the Trimurti or threefold powers in the universe: creation (Brahma), preservation (Vishnu), and transformation (Shiva). Simply put, it means "the All."

The verbal and auditory dimension of meditation reflects these objectives. In some approaches, they are regarded as powerful as other meditative activities such as breathing, posture, and mental exercises. Most associate the different forms of meditation sounds with mantra ("word"), the Yogic science of evoking conditions in the meditator through recitations. Just say the word, and you're there!

How Mantras Work

In the Middle East, you will hear the call to prayer five times a day. In Europe, the church bells sound daily. At Japanese shrines, wind chimes produce soothing sounds. In these cultures, sounds both awaken the listener and prepare for quieter moments, reminding everyone that peaceful times are approaching.

When entering into a meditation, we must first empty ourselves of thought. Reciting mantras and toning sounds facilitates this process. Repetitive auditory signals, especially if they are produced in a calming, consistent manner, relax thought. Then, launching into stillness requires less effort. It's important to remember that the science of mantra is a tool of meditation, but it is not meditation. Only when the mind is still is one in a state of meditation.

Meditative Toning

Mantras are often linked to vowels that resonate with the hearer in a comfortable, familiar way. Some suggest that the first vowel in your name is the most effective to use in meditation. This is because you are so used to hearing it that it is incorporated in your "vibration."

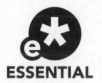

ESSENTIAL

Try an experiment to observe how sound affects the environment. Take a shallow dish and cover the surface with a small amount of water. Place the dish in front of a stereo speaker, turn on the music, and watch the patterns form on the surface. You'll notice different patterns forming when the musical rhythms and tones change.

There are many sounds that can be used to achieve balance and calm. Toning is one technique that is widely used for meditative and healing work. Toning is really an ancient art form, used to restore "harmonic balance" when illness or other crises occur. As with meditations practiced in many traditions, repetitiveness is important. The practitioner intones specific sounds repetitively, giving great care to quality and duration of the intonation. Think of it as mindful humming, though the mouth is not closed in this technique.

Vowel	Linked to
A (aah)	Relaxation, quiet
E (aay)	Humor, acceptance
I (eeh)	Stimulation, attention
O (ooh)	Concentration, focus
U (uuh)	Empathy, harmony

In this system, consonants have highlighting effect; in the same way punctuation gives meaning to the written word. For example, the *Om* mantra combines the focus of the *o* sound with the quality of extension provided by the *m* sound. In this way, words in prayer and meditation have become incorporated in the science of sacred language. While the Hindus resonate to *Om*, Christians and Jews use "Amen," and Muslims use *Amin*.

FACT

Researchers have discovered that a natural healing mechanism accounts for the purring sound of cats. The typical housecat rumbles on at a frequency of 27 to 44 hertz, while the puma, ocelot, and cheetah resonate at 20 to 50 Hz. These sounds promote the healing process in feline bones. And most amazingly, human exposure to such sound frequencies improves bone density.

Mantras to Use in Meditation

Sequences of words are also used in meditation to evoke particular states of awareness. Each tradition has its own powerful mantras, although some mantras may be used for specific circumstances. To use them, follow these guidelines:

1. Confine your use of mantras to one per meditation session.
2. Intone the mantra after you are physically settled; this sets the stage for evoking the particular state you are seeking.
3. Breathe in, then recite the mantra slowly while exhaling; intone each vowel for as long as possible, and use the consonants as "punctuation."
4. Recite the mantra three times, followed by two to three minutes of silence.
5. You may repeat this cycle as many times as you wish, but devote some time, at least ten to fifteen minutes, to conclude in silence and allow the mantra to vibrate within.

Here are some mantras with pronunciation keys:

- *Yod He Vau He* (yahd-hey-vow-hey): Hebrew, the holy name of God written as *YHWH* or "Jehovah."
- *Sat Nam* (saaht-namm): Yoga, "I am truth."
- *Om Mani Padme Hum* (ah-um-ma-nee-pad-may-hum): Buddhist, "Behold, the jewel in the lotus."

The Sound of Meditation

In ancient Greek mythology, Orpheus possessed a magical lyre made from an ox skull, with seven strings. Each of the strings was tuned to the motion of the seven planets and could induce the listener to hear the "music of the spheres." It is said that all who heard the sounds of this lyre—animals, planets, people, and even the elements—were transported to divine states of mind.

FACT

In an effort to see if there is a "God-oriented" part of the brain, researchers have attempted to track brain activity during meditation. The images resulting from these tests show diminished activity in the parietal lobe, where we orient ourselves in three-dimensional space and possess the sense of self. When this function is reduced, it appears that the boundary between the individual and the universe is also reduced.

Throughout time, some instruments have been associated with prayer and meditation. These instruments can be used to expand your practice and experience something new. It's a good idea to experiment with the sounds produced by these tools before you buy them, though. Most stores will not object to you listening for a time to the tones of an instrument you are considering for purchase. You might also listen to recorded music produced with certain instruments beforehand. If they help settle you mentally or emotionally, they will probably be helpful in your meditation oasis as well. Some instruments may be distracting to you. For example, the drum is very centering for bodywork, but distracting in mental exercises. Meditation instruments should be used to "set the stage" for a meditative session. They can be used to open a sitting that will be followed by silence, or a session can alternate between sound exercises and silent meditation. Here, it is just as important to discern the effects of sound following the experience of it. Instruments to consider include:

- **Drum:** Drums serve to maintain a consistent rhythm and work very well on the physical level, symbolizing the heartbeat. Rattles, shakers, and other percussion instruments work well, too.

- **Bell:** There are so many variations on bell tones that you should choose carefully. Bells are associated with the mental level and symbolize the breath.
- **Chimes:** Chimes are associated with the emotional level and symbolize the sense of touch. The flute and other wind instruments work well, too.
- **Singing Bowls:** Singing bowls are found in unique places, from Tibetan monasteries to South American temples. They may be metal or quartz crystal, and they "sing" or hum when skimmed with a wood or metal wand. Singing bowls are associated with the inspirational level and symbolize the sense of hearing.

Musical Chakras

A number of systems have been proposed that associate musical notes with the chakras or body centers. This is because a traditional practice in Yoga is to use meditation to energize the chakras in order to assist in therapeutic processes and overall balance.

To experience this form of meditation, begin in complete silence for about five minutes. You may use a visual of the chakras as they are aligned from bottom to top of the spinal column.

Beginning with the first chakra, and progressing upward, intone the *bija*, or sound of each center. The sounds and keys for each chakra are as follows:

1. *Lam*, G
2. *Vam*, A
3. *Ram*, B
4. *Yam*, C
5. *Ham*, D
6. *Om*, E
7. No sound, F

Intone slowly, first by inhaling and sounding the *bija* on exhalation. You may intone the *bija* for each chakra several times to focus on that center. Conclude by intoning the sacred formula, *So Haam* (sew-haaamm), "I am that."

CHAPTER 17

Meditation Aids

The lore of gems, power objects, and scents are age-old traditions that are beloved in both the East and West. They are closely associated with meditation by virtue of their alleged ability to influence both the meditator and the environment. What are you supposed to do with these objects? Are they valuable in meditation or are they just superstitious baubles?

Sacred Materials

Many cultures believe that natural objects can awaken special states of mind. This is not because the object itself has any power. Rather, the object is believed to "carry" certain powers that nature or human beings place into it. Many materials also have the weight of tradition behind them, and using the "right" materials shows deference or respect for those who have gone before.

In Buddhist cultures, there is a set of powerful gems and metals that the practitioner may present at the shrine. They are the *Sapta Ratnani* ("previous seven") of gold, silver, lapis lazuli, moonstone or crystal, agate, ruby or pearl, and carnelian. Each represents the aim of purifying the meditator's chakras as a gift to the Buddha. Likewise Native Americans assemble "medicine bags" that contain objects in nature that connect the holder to spiritual forces. They may include rare stones, the bones of animals, and bundles of dried herbs. The following sections cover three types of power objects that reflect such purposes: amulets, talismans, and relics.

ESSENTIAL

Your meditation oasis can feature any number of amulets, talismans, or relics. They can hang in a special place on the wall or be placed by a window to catch the wind and light. They serve as reminders of the special qualities you are striving for.

Amulets

Amulets are objects worn or carried to protect the individual from negative influences or to bring positive energies. These objects are derived from natural locales, sacred sites, or places where a divine presence has entered the environment. They are usually hard substances, such as bone, glass, metals, gems, stones, shells, and pottery. Amulets may be engraved or enclosed in a metal bezel.

Talismans

These objects do not occur naturally and they may carry an inscription, sigil, or design. Talismans may be made of paper or leather and bear a sacred name, form, or image of a divine force. They may be used to effect special circumstances or events for the wearer or carrier. In Japan, an individual may go to a Buddhist shrine and get an *Omamori* for a special goal. It's a tiny wooden tablet, placed in a silk bag and worn during meditation. Roman Catholics often wear scapulars to honor saints and to acquire their good qualities and protection through prayer.

Relics

These objects are the remains of holy persons or places. They may include pieces of clothing, hair, or bone, objects used by the person, or remains of a sacred building. The life force that once embodied relics is believed to still remain in them, providing healing or wisdom to the owner. In Catholic and Orthodox practice, relics are kept in a reliquary at a home or church altar. They serve as reminders of the grace that is transferred from the original source to a person through prayer. Mementos from deceased family or friends serve a similar purpose. They remind us of the heritage we wish to preserve.

Gems

Gems and semiprecious stones have a mythological character that is regarded as important to the wearer in many cultures. The belief in birthstones is part of this; it comes from the ancient art of astrology. Birthstones are supposed to transform the inherent weaknesses of each sign in the zodiac and bring out its strengths at the same time. For example, the Cancer native is subject to shifting moods, but the moonstone reflects serenity when it is needed.

Certain moods and states of mind are associated with precious stones. Whether worn or placed in the meditation environment, they are often regarded as important ways to balance and focus the mind and emotions. Gemstones are also associated with the chakras, and the wearing of them is alleged to balance their activity.

Gem	Mental Quality	Chakra
Amethyst	Wisdom	*Svadhisthana*
Diamond	Fortitude	*Sahasrara*
Emerald	Compassion	*Manipura*
Ruby	Devotion	*Vissuddha*
Sapphire	Integrity	*Ajna*
Selenite	Intuition	*Muladhara*
Topaz	Knowledge	*Anahata*

To the Greeks, the *ametho* (amethyst) is the "preventer of drunkenness." It is believed to protect the wearer against confusion and invites clear thinking. The Chinese believe that jade comes from the bones of dragons. The smooth green variety is believed to possess the five cardinal virtues: charity, modesty, wisdom, justice, and courage. The Native Americans of the southwestern United States believe that turquoise has numerous healing powers, so they fashion it into jewelry to protect the wearer from illness. If the stone cracks, they believe that the residing spirit has departed after absorbing the disease intended for the wearer.

Throughout history, various kinds of stones have been regarded as possessing healing powers. The belief has become transposed in some mindbody practices, such as healing and meditation.

FACT

According to biblical accounts, Aaron the brother of Moses was a high priest. Part of his regalia was a breastplate embedded with twelve stones, which symbolized the twelve tribes of Israel. Many relate this also to the twelve astrological signs, but whatever the association, the breastplate supposedly endowed special powers when worn.

In the Yogic science of Ayurveda, a repertoire of eighty-four gems is used to assist healing by enhancing certain energies. The Ayurvedic physician often recommends either wearing the gems or using them to make "gem waters." The gems are placed in water to rest for a time, and then the patient drinks the water for medicinal purposes. Medieval European physicians used the same procedure.

In meditation, the *navratnas,* or nine healing gems, are used to awaken the body's innate healing powers. The process begins with meditation, followed by visualization of the gem's healing colors and recitation of the planetary mantras that awaken the gem's energies. The meditator then wears the gem to help in the healing process.

Navratna	Energy	Mantra
Cat's-eye	Discrimination, self-knowledge	*Aum Kaim Ketave Namah Aum*
Coral	Determination, purpose	*Aum Bhaum Bhaumaye Namah Aum*
Diamond	Harmony, creativity	*Aum Shum Shu Kraye Namah Aum*
Emerald	Self-confidence, problem-solving	*Aum Bum Budhaye Namah Aum*
Lapis lazuli	Preservation	*Aum Sham Shanaish Charaya Namah Aum*
Pearl	Peace, comfort, intuition	*Aum Som Somaye Namah Aum*
Ruby	Vitality, resistance, immunity	*Aum Hring Hamsah Suryaye Namah Aum*
Sapphire	Truthfulness, charity	*Aum Brum Brahaspataye Namah Aum*
Zircon	Muscular strength	*Aum Ram Rahuye Namah Aum*

Crystals

In the late nineteenth century, Jacques and Pierre Curie discovered the phenomenon of piezoelectricity. They found that some crystals, particularly those derived from quartz, rapidly expand and contract on a molecular level when placed in alternating electrical fields. The reverse also occurs when crystals are placed in sound wave chambers, where they create electrical potentials or voltages. Because of this ability, piezoelectric crystals can be used as either receivers or sources of sound waves in acoustics. The sound waves can run the range of audible to ultrasonic frequencies.

So metaphysically, crystals—like other material that comes from the depth of the earth—are believed to embody and transmit the subtler frequencies in the environment. For the meditator, this can be beneficial, especially when crystals are placed in the meditation oasis. The frequencies that may be received from, for example, the long-term repetition of mantras, or the harmonic atmosphere of serenity, are "stored" in the crystal. It becomes a sort of organic record of meditative experience. At the same time, the crystal may influence the meditator to become "tuned" to the same atmosphere with less effort. Raw rock crystal is reported to be the most effective for this purpose.

Other types of crystal are also used in the meditation environment. Rose quartz is associated with the fourth chakra (love and devotion) and amethyst, a form of quartz, with the second chakra (wisdom and intuition). Manufactured lead crystal is also used to deter harmful influences, much in the same way that the *Pa Kua* is used in *feng shui*.

FACT

In the story of the Magi, the three kings traveled to Bethlehem from far-off countries, seeking the newborn Jesus. Many see parallels in this story, the gifts being akin to the "three jewels" of Buddhism. Melchior, king of Nubia, presented gold for "kingship"; Balthazar, king of Chaldea, presented frankincense for "devotion"; and Gaspar, king of Ethiopia, presented myrrh for "sacrifice."

Beads

Just about every culture has a custom of using beads in meditation or prayer. They help the user to focus on recitation and counting. The latter is itself a meditation, since counting breaths and figures within mandalas is an attentive mental exercise. Beads are usually held in one hand and counted with the thumb and forefinger. They also have the advantage of keeping the hands busy for people who tend to fidget. If not touched in sequence, the beads can be rubbed together by the meditator to stimulate attention. Ceremonial beads include:

- **Rosary:** Used for Catholic prayer, the rosary consists of five sets of beads, each consisting of ten small beads and one larger. These sets are joined in a loop by a crucifix. An Anglican version uses four sets of seven "week" beads with four "cruciform" beads marking the four directions.

- **Muslim Prayer Beads:** These prayer beads are used to silently recite the ninety-nine names of God. The ninety-nine beads are joined in a loop by a tassel.
- *Mala:* In Hindu and Buddhist meditation, 108 beads are strung together. Some *mala* are fabricated from sandalwood, which can be infused with scented oils. In the yogic tradition, rudraksha ("Rudra's tears") and tulasi ("holy basil") beads are used.
- **Chinese Meditation Balls:** The two metal balls fit into the palm of the hand and resonate musically when moved around by the fingers. They are a good choice for concentrating exercise and are believed to harmonize the meditator with sounds when used consistently.
- **Prayer Stones:** The cool feeling of these rounded stones, also called touch stones, can be relaxing. They can be carried outside of the meditation oasis to the office desk or dentist's chair as psychic reinforcement for calm.

The Science of Smell

The sense of smell is one of the most powerful instruments we possess to connect the outer world with inner states. Scent is inhaled through the nose, traveling through the olfactory nerves into receptors in the brain. From there, scent creates changes in the limbic system, a primitive area in the brain that governs emotions and memory. It is through this simple act of inhaling that molecules of scent can impact our psychological state.

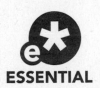

ESSENTIAL

Scientists have recorded hundreds of emotional responses to the scents of flowers, herbs, and other organic materials. As a result, aromatherapy has become widely popular because it features a natural approach to understanding the realms of thought and feeling. The meditation culture has also embraced aromatherapy as an important adjunct to practice.

In the 1970s, Robert Tisserand, a researcher in the science of smell, produced a body of work inspired by the studies of Dr. Jean Valnet in France. Tisserand demonstrated the tremendous influence and potential of aromatic plants for the health of body and mind. His was one of the first expositions on the science of aromatherapy, which now has become a buzzword in everyday business and leisure. Tisserand made the connection between aromatic substances and the human endocrine system. In addition, studies he observed showed that scent could actually alter brain-wave activity.

FACT

The ability of a scent to attract the attention and interest of a subject is based on its concentration of pheromones (from the Greek, "to transfer excitement"). Pheromones are complex molecular structures that transmit signals through the air via scent. Animals and insects have it, and humans do, too. Pheromones play a considerable role in creating the magnetic attraction between the sexes.

Marketers have long since known about the power of smell to seduce customers, and the field of aromatherapy is rapidly developing scent for healing. A Japanese website has started mapping unusual scents around the world so that aficionados can sample them. In 2009 at Brigham Young University, researchers found that smells associated with cleanliness (in this case, citrus-scented Windex) led test subjects to reciprocate trust. Take some of this wisdom into your practice space: keep it clean and lightly scented with something calming and inspiring.

Mood Mapping with Scent

Scent is big business. Scientists who specialize in understanding the effects of scent on mood and mind are called odorologists. In recent years, odorologists have been investigating which smells influence states of mind in order to create a "mood map" that reveals the secrets of scent. Preliminary results show that citrus is mentally stimulating, vanilla is relaxing, and rose is calming. For therapeutic use, odorologists have confirmed that cucumber helps claustrophobics.

And that's not all. The presence of certain smells can influence performance. Experiments have shown that children test better in school with floral scents in the atmosphere, while adults exercise harder (without noticing it) when strawberry is released into the environment. One of the more interesting developments is research in Japan on weight loss using scent. Researchers at Shiseido, a well-respected cosmetics giant, are releasing a body lotion that they claim will stimulate the brain to discharge hormones that burn fat. Some of the ingredients they have disclosed are grapefruit and pepper. Other studies show the scents of apple and banana have a similar effect on test subjects who are dieting.

Department stores have caught on to this phenomenon and use it extensively. To stimulate customer interest and patronage, stores are releasing scents through potpourri "cookers," ventilation systems, and old-fashioned spray bottles.

It's important to be aware of these trends. Scent has always been known to have a subliminal effect, and in recent times this knowledge has been confirmed by science. As a result, fragrance is used even more to influence our thinking and moods. A positive way to counter the trend is to use scent in meditation, when our senses are functioning optimally. By wisely choosing fragrances that support the meditative environment and our own goals, we may become the cartographers of our own mood maps.

The Soul of Meditation

In the Middle East, perfume is regarded as the "soul" of the plant; for the French, scent is the music of the senses. When mosques were built in the Middle Ages, the mortar was mixed with rose oil, so the walls would exude a divine odor at midday. In a similar way, we can use scent to evoke moods that support meditation. While doing this, the innate healing qualities of certain scents can also assist in physical and emotional well-being.

ALERT

Incense burners and potpourri bowls heated with candles should be used with caution. Choose terracotta, clay, stone, or metal holders that have ample room to catch the ashes. Incense wands last a little more than half an hour, which is also a good way to time a meditation session.

In your meditation oasis, you may use items that provide a continuous scented atmosphere. There are hot and cold diffusers, which require an electrical outlet to operate. Scented oils or waters are placed in a receptacle that releases the mist in timed or graduated amounts. Choose one that will shut off automatically when emptied. You can also moderate the scented atmosphere on your own by using spray bottles whenever you choose. In that way, you can alternate different scents as a "sense exercise." Just be sure to point spray bottles away from the walls and furniture when you use them.

Incorporating incense into your meditation brings the "soul" of contemplation into the atmosphere. Entering a room where incense has been burning can instantly place you in a relaxed zone. Even the residue of incense is calming, as it penetrates furniture, curtains, and even pet fur.

Burned Offerings

In ancient Mexico, the Maya manufactured and traded incense in great quantities. Copal incense, taken from a variety of Central American pine trees, was believed to purify the dwelling. It was also pressed into cakes decorated with the heads of their deities and carried through crop fields to sanctify them.

FACT

When a British monarch is crowned, a traditional oil—said to include benzoin, rose, cinnamon, jasmine, musk, civet, and ambergris—is created for anointing the royal person into power. Pouring it on the head of the monarch repeats a tradition that goes back to ancient Egypt and the days of King Solomon. The powers of the oil are believed to "awaken" the monarch's royal intelligence.

Native North Americans also purify spaces with dried herbs. Small bundles of cedar, tobacco, sweet grass, and sage are burned and used to "smudge" windows and doors to prevent harmful influences from entering a sacred space. Incense imparts a feeling of the sacred and can support the atmosphere of meditation. Here are some suggestions for incense selections:

- **For facilitating breath work during pranayama:** Eucalyptus, pine, and lavender are clean and penetrating scents.
- **For mental focus:** Basil, geranium, and frankincense penetrate deeply through the emotional sphere and have lasting power.
- **For purifying emotions:** Jasmine, vetiver, sage, and cypress have a calming effect on mood.
- **For neutralizing stress:** Rosemary reduces melancholy, and scents of the mint family (peppermint, spearmint) are mentally uplifting.
- **For an inspirational atmosphere:** Patchouli, sandalwood, and myrrh are the traditional ingredients for liturgical incense.

The Merits of Incense

Japanese culture places KŌ ("incense") high on the list of meditative elements. Like tea, which was brought into Japan in the sixth century, incense is regarded as a sacred substance. During the Edo period, the art of *Kodo,* the "Way of Incense," arose. It is a process of "listening" to the delicate scent of incense as it burns. An event similar to the tea ceremony is arranged, in which fragrant substances are burned for reflection. The classical Japanese story, *The Tale of Genji,* speaks of this art eloquently: The Ten Virtues of Burning KŌ are as follows:

- Incense opens the mind to divinity.
- Incense cleanses the mind.
- Incense divests the mind of worldly impurities.
- Incense awakens the mind.
- Incense encourages the mind in solitude.
- Incense affords the mind leisure when it is busy.
- Even a little incense is not enough.

- Age does not affect the efficacy of incense.
- Habitual use of incense causes no harm.

Meditation Oils

In some meditation systems, to enhance mental clarity and emotional balance, the practitioner anoints his or her body with essential plant oils. Certain scents protect, purify, elevate feeling, and repel negative thoughts, and certain parts of the body correlate to these functions:

- **Brow:** The intuitive sense
- **Crown:** The mental processes
- **Feet:** Purification for healing, trauma
- **Hands:** To bring grace to one's work following meditation
- **Heart:** The emotional plane
- **Solar plexus:** The physical functions

A Catalog of Scent

To be most effective, essential oils should be pure and uncut. Oils should never be kept in plastic containers. Traditionally, essential oils are stored in amber or blue glass to protect them from ultraviolet light. They should be touched on the body with cotton or an eyedropper, since placing the fingers directly on the bottle opening can alter the purity of the scent within.

Oil	Use
Cedar	Dispels sluggishness, lethargy
Cinnamon	Treats fatigue, depression
Eucalyptus	Has a cooling influence; helps with anger
Frankincense	Maintains meditation focus; inspirational and rejuvenating
Geranium	Has an uplifting vibration; addresses anxiety
Jasmine	"Softens" the emotions; treats listlessness, fear
Lavender	Aids memory and alleviates mental stress; old-fashioned headache remedy
Neroli (orange blossom)	Counters insomnia, nervous tension
Patchouli	Clarifies problems; encourages objectivity
Pine	Lessens claustrophobia; elevates emotions
Rose	Functions as an antidepressant; effective for grief

Oil	Use
Sage	Supports healing processes, the purification of space
Sandalwood	Evokes confidence and supports meditation overall; revered in Ayurveda

The Power of Plants

Herbalism and phytotherapy (curing with plants) are among the many vital fields of healing research. The preference of many people for natural approaches drives much of this, along with the growing acceptance that plants are more than stems, roots, and seeds. Laboratory experiments conducted over the past three decades, suggest that plants have some form of consciousness and react to sound—from music to the human voice.

We all know someone who has a "green thumb." He seems to be able to grow anything effortlessly and his home is filled with delightful plants and flowers. What may distinguish these people from the rest of us who labor over scrawny little vines is the ability to become meditative with the plant. How is this done? Most gardeners will agree that when you become involved with the growing, feeding, and caring of a plant, you establish a subtle relationship with it. And in that relationship there isn't much room for your own thoughts and feelings. There is only the soil, water, and the seed.

QUOTE

"When you find your soul, you will bloom where you are planted."

—Anonymous

Working with nature in this way is an exercise that removes you from the constraints of time. The rhythm of planting, nurturing, and watching the plant grow and yield its benefits is timeless because it's always going on around us. Becoming part of that rhythm is rather effortless, too. It's really just a matter of finding your plant soul.

Finding Your Plant Soul

Just as there are as many meditation styles as there are people, so there are plants for everyone who wants to experience this relationship with nature. You can find the type of plant that resonates to your personality and subtly imparts its qualities to you and your meditation environment.

Look at plant and flower catalogs to learn something about their care. At the same time, study the photographs of the mature plants and make note of the colors and types that appeal to you. Consider some basics of what you want from the plant. Will it be culinary (to eventually eat), functional (to provide oxygenation or ward off insects), or decorative? Balance the basics with the subtle qualities the plant can provide: scent, color, a feeling of calm, healing, beauty.

Start out with just a few growing things in your meditation environment. If they become prolific, all your meditation time may wind up being devoted to their care.

Experience the plants and flowers directly. Visit nurseries, flower shows, and public gardens. Ask the caretakers about plant qualities they have learned from experience. If a particular plant appeals to you, spend some time looking at it and reflecting on its qualities. Be attentive; you may get a response.

If looking after plants is not your idea of a meditative practice, consider other things that can grow in your environment. Mosses convey the image of time in slow motion and of old forests; small trees can be starters for your future landscape projects. Zen gardens that feature only rock and sand landscapes can be just as calming as living plants.

CHAPTER 18

In Celebration of Life

Many people complain that the absence of ritual in our modern life results in a feeling of emptiness. Weddings and baptisms, wakes and funerals—all of these are rituals that assist us in coping with fear and change in varying degrees. We often dismiss them as unimportant or time-consuming, forgetting that ritual is a vital component in every culture. Ritual makes the ordinary sacred.

Everyday Rituals

Having rituals in your life doesn't mean taking part in elaborate ceremonies with special robes and chamber music. When you think about it, there are thousands of rituals that form a part of everyday life. Brushing your teeth, walking the dog, even the way you eat meals—these activities all incorporate ritual behavior. They are rituals because you repeat certain actions when you perform the task and you never deviate from those actions because they have meaning for you. You may have developed these rituals on your own, out of necessity and preference. Or some rituals may have been imposed on you, by custom or family influence.

QUOTE

"We worship Agni, the fire god,
He who always does good for others,
As progenitor of seasons and beholder of gems."
—The Rig-Veda (ancient collection of Hindu sacred verses)

Can everyday rituals be sacred? Yes, they can be filled with meaning when they are performed meditatively. By focusing our attention on ordinary acts that we usually perform without thinking, we can learn a great deal. We can discover why certain actions that we repeat are so meaningful. Here are some examples of ordinary rituals: You always fold your laundry in neat little bundles. When you polish a mirror, you use only one cleaner and work from top to bottom. When watching television, you always groom your fingernails.

These revelations can be sacred because everyday acts can reflect your motives, feelings, and goals in life—in essence, everything that you are. The key to engaging this process is to employ a meditative attitude in all those little rituals. In our example, a meditative attitude that is engaged while you are performing these tasks could reveal the following: There was a time when you had little space of your own. Folding your laundry in little bundles was a way to get all your laundry put away in the space you had. You fondly remember a grandparent who polished a mirror the same way. You miss that person a great deal. It's important that you not waste spare time, so grooming while watching television takes care of two things at once.

You can take this attentiveness another step and make these little rituals more meaningful. If you now have plenty of living space, you could make a ritual out of decorating and appreciating it. You could honor a beloved relative by creating a home gallery of family pictures for a weekly ritual of remembrance. You could make a ritual out of grooming with all your attention focused on yourself.

The objective here is to recognize that rituals have meaning. When you discover that, you are opening the treasure trove of your memories, talents, and repressed needs.

Social Rituals

Social rituals are inevitable and they dictate a great deal of our public lives. You are never alone here; these rituals involve family, coworkers, and community members. There is usually a protocol to these events, and very little room for spontaneity. Some are events that you may look forward to; others you may dread because you'll have to interact with people you don't like. However, they are opportunities to understand others and find a meeting of ideas and feelings.

ESSENTIAL

Socializing is important, but the ritual that makes it possible has meaning. When you participate in social rituals wholeheartedly, you influence those around you to take notice of the meaning as well.

One way to inject meaning into these situations is, once again, to become aware of the ritual and of those who are participating. If you just go through the motions mindlessly, everyone will go away with relief that it's over and lose out on an opportunity to relate in a meaningful way.

Be conscious of everyone who is present. In Zen monasteries, the monks offer a form of thanksgiving at each meal: "Sixty-four pairs of hands brought this meal to the table." It's an acknowledgment of the community effort required to accomplish a single task.

In a clockwise direction, scan the room or space you're in, and make note of each person. Include the hosts, the guests, and the staff. Observe the uniqueness of each person. Acknowledge each person's presence in the room, verbally or with your body language (waving, nodding, smiling directly at the person).

Participate in the ritual fully. If, for example, it is an awards ceremony, applaud those being honored. If it's a memorial service, reflect on the memories being recalled. If it is a religious service, aim to perform your part flawlessly.

Don't act distracted or give the impression you are busy (making calls on your cell phone) or impatient (looking at a watch or clock), or are thinking of someone else you would rather see. Afterward, acknowledge the contributions of the other participants. Let them know how meaningful their words and actions are to you.

Business Rituals

When you purchase a house, the closing is a ritual that requires you, your attorney, real estate agent, and a host of other "officials" to be present and follow a protocol that seems like a terrible waste of time. But try to talk the participants out of it and you'll be surprised at how stubbornly they insist on following the prescribed order of things.

Business meetings are another dilemma. Certainly, problems have to be solved and agreements have to be made. But the rituals involve everything from political maneuvering to departmental competition.

When you're in a business meeting, acknowledge everyone's effort to come together and address the present situation. Have a pleasant expression. Give encouragement; unify everyone's thinking by emphasizing points that all agree upon. Maintain a mindful posture without slumping or sprawling.

Be attentive; don't tap your pencil, turn pages, or fidget. Let each speaker know she has your full attention. Breathe evenly.

Show compassion; point out each individual's abilities to resolve a particular issue. Discourage stress by finding ways those present can reflect on solving knotty problems rather than come up with instantaneous solutions.

Meditation Rituals

Ritual serves a sublime purpose. Sociologists like it because it keeps us in the community flow. Therapists suggest it for overcoming grief. Meditators see it as valuable because it gives meaning to ordinary action.

Ideally, ritual should nurture our individuality and provide us a means to express it in ways of our own choosing. Many traditional cultures offer ways to do this, from maintaining personal shrines at home to going on prayer pilgrimages to sacred places. But in the quiet of your own space, you can design rituals that place you in the meditative spirit. Such rituals let you perform symbolic acts (causes) to elicit desired results (effects). It is the basis of what is regarded as sympathetic magic, but it is grounded in meditative action because it uses the same faculties as meditation: attention, awareness, and visualization.

A Candle Meditation

Candles have become a popular way to scent living space and add festivity to a gathering. You can find just about any size, shape, color, or fragrance to complement your décor. For meditation practice, candles can also provide an atmosphere that supports your intentions. In addition, they offer their own little rituals that reflect your goals.

Choose a candle color that reflects your intentions. Choose a scent that embodies your goals. Devote a full session to the candle meditation. Dim the lights, but avoid a completely dark room.

Begin by assembling candle(s), matches or lighter, candleholder(s), and snuffer. Use a separate table or stand for the candle.

Allow yourself five minutes to attain even breathing and physical composure. As you are doing this, close your eyes and think of your mind as a candle, awaiting illumination.

Strike the match or lighter with a flourish. Keep your eyes on the flame as you light the candle. Gaze at the flame and think of it as the spirit of illumination that is lighting your mind. Give yourself twenty-five minutes to gaze. When you put out the candle, do so deliberately. Understand that the spirit of illumination can enter your life whenever you give it attention by lighting the candle.

Ritual and Analytic Psychology

In the early twentieth century, the eminent Swiss psychologist Carl Gustav Jung broke away from his brilliant mentor, Sigmund Freud. Jung strongly disagreed with the founder of psychoanalysis on several points. But one of the most important issues, Jung argued, was that human instinct is not based in death and sexuality alone. He proposed that the experience of spirit is also a fundamental drive in human nature. Jung spent the rest of his life pursuing as many facets of that view as possible, and his legacy has enriched our understanding of the inner life in a multitude of ways.

Jung explored alchemy, religion, mystical symbolism, astrology, shamanism, and all of the meditation systems we have examined. In them, he discovered keys that offer positive transformation of the human condition that have been revered through the ages—including reflection, prayer, ritual, and group participation. As a result of those studies, Jung developed an approach to understanding the inner life that doesn't limit our experience to thinking and feeling. Instead, he considered all our dimensions, including intuition, sensation, and creativity. Working on these levels includes dreams, visions, work, play, art, and ritual.

Jung pointed out that ritual experience is a powerful tool for transformation. Through it, the process of individuation ("becoming individualized") can take place. This wisdom is imparted in many meditation traditions. The Japanese tea ceremony is both a meditation and a social ritual, while Native American drumming is more than making music. Both are means of focusing attention and leaving ordinary reality for the realm of spirit. The conscious act of performing these rituals focuses attention, energy, and the ego into the pure act of doing.

Jung's work coalesced into the practice of analytic psychology. Meditation is an approach deeply entwined in the process, because it allows the inner dimensions of the person to come forward. Analytic psychology also encourages the use of traditional symbols because they have universal meaning.

Five Elements Meditation

In Yogic philosophy, the five elements are known as the *tattwas*. They are the embodiments of the universal forces: fire, earth, air, water, and *akasha* (spirit). When these forces are in balance, there is harmony. Rest (earth) and activity (fire) are in unison, as are thought (air) and feeling (water). Together, they allow for creation (*akasha*) to proceed.

The creative impulse can enliven your work, play, and rest. That is why the Five Elements meditation is so useful and universal. Besides the Yogis, the Taoists, kabbalists, and Native Americans have some variation on it. It is symbolized in mandalas, with the four physical elements surrounding the fifth creative element in the center. It is also represented in the five sacred directions of many traditions.

▼ CHARACTERISTICS OF THE FIVE ELEMENTS

Element	Color	Figure	Vowel	Taoist Image	Yogic Stage	Instrument	Direction	Dimension
Fire	Red	Triangle	I	Phoenix	*Samadhi* (Being)	Gong	East	Intuition
Earth	Yellow	Square	O	Dragon	*Sushupti* (Deep sleep)	Drum	North	Sensation
Air	Blue	Circle	A	Tiger	*Jagrat* (Waking)	Harp	West	Thinking
Water	Green	Crescent	U	Tortoise	*Svapna* (Dreaming)	Bell	South	Feeling
Akasha	Violet	Oval	E	Serpent	*Avastha* (Enlightenment)	Rattle	Center	Creativity

The aim of this meditation is to balance the five dimensions—intuition, sensation, thinking, feeling, and creativity—within you. Draw or construct separate images of the elements on art board. *Akasha* should be placed in the center of the board. Above it, place water and below, earth. To the right of *akasha*, place fire, with air to the left. Using their associated colors adds to their efficacy. On the reverse, inscribe their corresponding attributes.

Place the images on a flat area of your meditation space according to their directional orientation (fire-east, water-south, air-west, earth-north, *akasha*-center). You are creating a three-dimensional mandala.

Sit before the mandala so that earth-north is right in front of you. Starting with fire-east (on your left) and moving in a clockwise direction, spend at least five minutes focused on each element.

You may gaze at each symbol in sequence, then close your eyes and evoke the symbol within your mind. Open your eyes and look at the symbol once more. Reverse each image and reflect on the information you have inscribed on the reverse. When you have completed the circle (east-south-west-north), go to the center and spend additional time on the symbol there.

African-American Meditation

The observance of Kwanzaa (Swahili for "fruits of the harvest") is a secular, African-American holiday developed in 1966 by Dr. Maulana Karenga. It is comprised of seven separate daily events that form a holiday in midwinter, from December 26 to January 1. This is a time in most cultures for reflecting and reformulating goals, when the days are shortest and light is minimal in the Northern Hemisphere. Most of the more profound ritual meditations take place at this time, reminding participants of the return of spring and the vitality it brings.

QUOTE

"Our Father, it is thy universe, it is thy will,
Let us be at peace,
Let the soul of thy people be cool.
Thou art our Father,
Remove all evil from our path."

—Nuer prayer, East Africa

The purpose of Kwanzaa is to honor the heritage and importance of family and community. At its core are seven principles called the *Nguzo Saba.* On each day of the cycle, one of the principles is recited and a candle is lighted to acknowledge and honor it as a goal. It is a marvelous combination of ritual meditation and affirmation. Here are the seven principles as recited by the participants:

1. **Umoja (unity):** To work together peacefully with our family, community, nation, and race.
2. **Kujichagulia (self-determination):** To make up our minds to accomplish the goals we have set for ourselves.
3. **Ujima (collective work and responsibility):** To team together and make our community a safe and productive place.
4. **Ujamaa (co-operative economics):** To build and maintain our own stores, shops, and other businesses, and profit from them together.
5. **Nia (purpose):** To have a plan for the future and be willing to help others to succeed.

6. **Kuumba (creativity):** To always do as much as we can, in any way we can, in order to leave our community a better and more beautiful place.
7. **Imani (faith):** To believe with all our heart in our people, our parents, our teachers, our leaders, and the righteousness and victory of our struggle.

Many African-Americans with ancestry from slaves keep a small home altar, often on a bench or stool, to honor their forebears. The altar may hold photographs or personal possessions of the previous generations, and, if the family practices African or Afro-Caribbean religions, perhaps ritual objects and images of deities. The shrine becomes a place to remember those who have died and carry their spirits into the future. If you have African ancestry, you may wish to set up your own shrine or explore African cultural associations in your area for more information. People of European ancestry can similarly inquire into their own ancestry and seek to make amends for European exploitation of African slaves. Making a donation to a scholarship fund or attending Martin Luther King, Jr. Day remembrance services can be a good start. The past shapes the present, and coming to grips with the past must happen for real transformation to take place.

The Moon and Meditation

In the early 1990s, British astronomer Dr. Percy Seymour sparked controversy in the scientific establishment by proposing that our brains are wired to the cycles of the Sun, the Moon, and the planets. Instead of repeating the simplistic view that these celestial bodies have a direct effect on us, he presented a more thought-provoking alternative. It is resonance, he said, that links us to the heavens. What this means is that we have a biochemical relationship to the celestial bodies, which links our own rhythms to their rhythmic cycles.

Seymour also pointed out that ancient people were more aware of changes in earth's electromagnetic field than we are today, and not because of evolution. Rather, it is our departure from nature, physically and mentally. Despite this, he argues, we still possess the ancient skills of "wayfinding," a sixth sense that recognizes the connection between human events and celestial ones.

Belief in a relationship between the stars and human life is as old as civilization. In fact, the concept of divine life has always been equated with the appearances of the sunrise, the full moon, and the passing of stars overhead.

FACT

Most of the world today holds some variation on the belief in astrology. Cultures associated with Buddhism, Hinduism, and Islam, as well as the beliefs of indigenous people around the world, have always held astrology in high esteem. Royal marriages and business enterprises—even political events and military coups—are still planned by the stars.

The Lunar Month

The sun and moon are the two luminaries in celestial science, because they reflect light to us on earth. In meditation, they represent the conscious mind (sun) and the inner, unconscious mind (moon). Through meditative experience, these two dimensions must reflect each other, and this is symbolized by the full moon. In Buddhist tradition, the Buddha was believed to have achieved enlightenment at the full moon in May, when the sun is traveling through the constellation of Taurus. Other cultures see the sun-moon relationship in a similar way. They are the visible manifestations of yin and yang in Taoism, and the turning of the soul (moon) toward God (sun) in Islam.

The lunar month begins at the new moon. The sun and moon are in the same place in the heavens at this time, and there is no moonlight in the night sky. Over the next fourteen days, the moon will increase (wax) in visible light, starting with a sliver and growing to a crescent. When the moon is seven days old, half of its face is visible; and when it is fourteen days old, its full face appears in the sky. Following this event, the moon will decrease (wane) in visible light. Its full face will gradually diminish over the next fourteen days to a half moon, and then a crescent. Eventually, the light will disappear and the cycle starts all over again with the next new moon.

Meditating with the Moon Phases

Being mindful of the Sun-Moon relationship can provide some interesting meditation experiences. You can also use the phases to time your goals and progress. For example, you can set a goal at the new moon and anticipate its accomplishment fourteen days later, at the full moon. Nearly every calendar provides a notation on the days of the lunar phases, and it is very easy to follow.

ESSENTIAL

A number of meditation systems use the lunar cycle as a timekeeping device. At the new moon, the meditator initiates a new program for self-awareness. At the first quarter, insights are sought. At the full moon, the meditator strives for understanding of what has been discovered. At the third quarter, there is introspection. And at the end of the cycle, when the moon has returned to darkness, the meditator "just sits."

New Moon

This is the beginning of the lunar cycle each month. In meditation, it is the beginning of a journey, entry onto a new path of experience. This is the time to draw attention to a new goal you may have initiated. Your attention should be sharp and limited to essentials. If you wish to break away from old patterns, this is the opportunity to start. Breathwork is a beneficial approach right now. Your meditation keywords are birth and beginnings.

First Quarter Moon

In this phase, results or feedback from your meditation work are forthcoming. As the Moon grows in light, so your self-awareness will increase. This is the time to increase your physical involvement in the meditation environment. Incorporate stretches before a session and change your posture in midsession. Your meditation keywords are growth and progress.

Full Moon

In this phase, illumination is indicated. Special insights may be forthcoming as you settle into a routine of stillness and observation. Professionals in the healing arts recognize that this lunar phase brings increased sensitivity, but your meditation work will prepare you for your increased perception of everything around you. Your meditation keywords are awareness and inspiration.

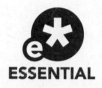

ESSENTIAL

Meditation groups find it useful to use the lunar cycle to coordinate sessions. It allows participants to make use of the visible rhythms in the sky and follow a nature-oriented practice.

Third Quarter Moon

With the diminishing light of the Moon, reflection is called for. In this phase your faculty of memory is highlighted, enabling you to recall thoughts and emotions with clarity. This is the phase of releasing and allowing your perceptions to float in stillness. Efforts you have made from the beginning of the cycle will bear fruit at this time. Your meditation keywords are realization and resolution.

Divination

Many people are attracted to divination because it offers the opportunity for reflection and self-awareness. Alone with a single question, your mind and emotions become focused on one point.

We have already looked at tarot cards, but there are many other forms of divination that have developed over time and around the world. The Northern cultures made great use of runes, small stones or animal bones inscribed with ancient alphabetic symbols. In China, the mystical oracle of the *I Ching* ("*Book of Changes*") brought guidance to unsettled questions. In other cultures, people perform mirror gazing or scrying for insight. These rituals use bowls of water or large stones (the original "crystal ball") to focus attention on the empty space of the mind.

Does this relate to meditation? Yes, because many of the techniques employed in meditation—such as stilling the mind and bringing the senses into focus—are required for a true divination. At the same time, certain methods of divination help develop intuition. Sometimes this is just a matter of confirming what you already know and realizing that it is a meditative experience.

Whatever your choice of divination—whether it's throwing coins, reading cards, counting sticks, or dropping stones—you will gain much from the experience if you use a meditative approach. For example, perform your divinations at your meditation oasis. The kitchen table or business desk is not conducive to meditative thought. Practice your breathing and body postures as if you were preparing for meditation. This will remove the anticipation and stress from your thinking and allow you to have an open mind. When you are clear, focus your thought on only the question that you want answered. Eliminate unnecessary thoughts about the situation, people, or conditions surrounding the question. Perform the divination without anticipating any answer. Record the answer or reading you receive and save it for a meditation session that may follow.

CHAPTER 19

Meditation in Motion

Although meditation aims for stillness and the quieting of the body and senses, it doesn't mean you have to just "sit" through it. We've seen how some meditation approaches make full use of the senses and our mobility. Moving meditations can make good use of the necessary—and pleasurable—tasks that fill our daily lives.

The Tiger and the Dragon

When Asian martial arts were initially divulged to the West in the twentieth century, most of their meditative roots remained hidden. Instead, the glamour of speed, precision, and the quiet little guy getting the best of the bully took center stage. Sure, we all knew there were "ancient Chinese secrets" to be learned, ones that could unlock the powers of combat and endurance. But we assumed that they were also techniques for using brute force and aggression, only in different ways than we used them in the West. Some films still reflect those assumptions, despite the accessibility of the metaphysical dimension in martial arts today.

In Asian culture, two consistent images present themselves to the practitioner as themes of the warrior nature: the tiger and the dragon.

The tiger is a highly reactive animal, instinctive and aggressive. It is relentless in its pursuit of prey and devastating when it has concluded the chase. All energy is expended in the hunt and the kill; then the animal is satiated and enters oblivion, in complete and unconscious rest. Because of its habits, the tiger lives a very short life.

The dragon is restful but observant. All energy is conserved. Its senses are engaged in the awareness of time, space, and everything that is within and around its existence. It does not hunt; it waits. When it encounters its prey, it allows the unconsciousness of the opponent (brought by fear or overconfidence) to do the work. Because of these habits, the dragon lives a very long life.

The warrior spirit is a necessary role in every life, and sometimes we are called on to assume it. If you are called to a combative situation, physical and mental preparation are absolutely necessary, but only meditation can engage the body and mind in taking the proper action. Here are some meditative points to cultivate:

- For the warrior, skill comes naturally and the ego is the only obstacle.
- Overcoming the ego, and not the opponent, is the mastery of the warrior.
- The ego is nourished by the emotions; by relinquishing fear, anger, and aggression, the mind becomes clear.
- When the mind is clear, appropriate action—defensive or offensive—can be taken.

- The peaceful warrior anticipates the outcome, not the process.
- The skillful warrior allows the opponent's emotions to work against him.
- The compassionate warrior cultivates a respect for self and for others.

Meditative Spirit and Team Sports

Sports usually involve groups of people and the formation of a team. And in most competitive sports, the team is the core of the game.

This is probably the toughest obstacle in sports. Relinquishing your individuality to become a part of something else, even if it's temporary and not binding, is a bigger challenge than having the skill to win at the game. For children, it's the best exercise for socializing the personality and civilizing the instincts. For adults, it's a hard task to give up an identity you've worked for years to create. But it's the only way to get the full reward of sports: achieving a flawless performance in unison with others.

The Meditative Team

Being involved with a team means building a group mind. One of the best ways to accomplish this is through group meditation, which bonds the minds of the individuals to create a team consciousness.

Individual members of the team should be knowledgeable and honest about their own strengths and weaknesses. They should also have the opportunity to communicate those strengths and weaknesses to the others. With an understanding and acceptance of those qualities, the goals of the team—to perform and compete well—are reinforced.

These points can be discussed; but to become truly meaningful, they should be included in group meditation sessions. The key strategies are releasing the individual ego and engaging the group mind. This process builds the inviolate circle of the team, what NBA coach Phil Jackson calls the "sacred hoop," a Lakota Sioux tribal concept.

When the time comes for playing the game, the group mind must be directed by a coach who possesses more than an awareness of the individual strengths and weaknesses. The potential of the whole to achieve goals and bringing the group mind to that awareness can be developed through group meditation.

The Meditative Athlete

There is some emphasis in sports circles on being "in the zone" of a game, completely absorbed in the play. This may well be a metaphor for blurring the ego enough to experience the rhythm of the event and the flow of the players together. But it is really moving meditation.

> "My first act after being named head coach of the Bulls was to formulate a vision for the team. I had learned from the Lakota and my own experience as a coach that vision is the source of leadership, the expansive dream state where everything begins and all is possible."
>
> —Phil Jackson, NBA Coach

The playing field is a mandala of experience. Your personal meditations should be focused on that mandala, and your experience should be in all parts of it. Whether your game gives you the opportunity to move through all the parts of the mandala, your bond with the group mind allows it to happen.

Winning is not the aim of your participation, becoming part of the flow is. Your responsibility to the game is to fuse with your team and play with one mind. Your reward from the team is the opportunity to play to your optimum ability.

Your Own Sacred Dance

Moving in a free flow is the objective of some meditative systems. Here, the mind is freed of thought when the body is freed of its inhibitions and everyday habits. Dance has always been a vehicle for this experience. It is one of the few meditative activities that allow for self-expression. This is because the body possesses all the natural rhythms needed to blend with the larger and subtler life rhythms around us.

In Hawaii, where much of the ancient culture still lives despite the incursion of colonialism, the indigenous dance tradition lives through the *hula halau* ("dance house"). Many think of Hawaiian dance as touristy performances, but the *kahiko hula* ("ancient dance") is a powerfully expressive moving meditation. It combines poetry, chant, religious symbolism, and movement in the body of the dancer.

The Hawaiians see the human body as having three *pikos* (navels). The first is at the crown of the head; it connects us to the past, to our ancestors. The second, in the middle of the torso, connects us to the present, to our parents and siblings. The third, at the genitals, connects us to our children, the future. In the body of the dancer, these three navels connect to the stream of life and are joined in rhythm.

We can easily follow the thinking of cultures like the Hawaiians' in using dance to join the body with the dimensions we are separate from. Like them, we can be aware of the connections we have to the different streams of life: past, present, and future. We can also be mindful of the different realms in which we move: body, mind, spirit. And we can do all of this by evoking the meditative attitude.

If you want to practice meditative dance, arrange your space so there is unobstructed room to move. Choose music that you personally feel resonance with. Rhythm is more important than style or lyrics. Choose an instrument that you can play to accompany the music, if possible. Bells, chimes, drums, or any percussion are simple to incorporate into dance.

FACT

Originating in ancient China, *yu pu* is a meditative dance performed by Taoist masters. Its purpose is to attract beneficial spirits while driving away harmful ones. The dance resembles a slow, limping gait that imitates birds walking among pebbles.

Spend at least fifteen minutes in a warm-up that should include breathing exercises for oxygenation and Yoga stretches to limber and tone muscles. Listen to the music during your warm-up to become accustomed to the rhythm.

Begin with at least fifteen minutes of simple movement. Swaying and turning in the beginning; then rhythmically moving your feet, arms, and hands. Use as much of your body as possible. See the musical rhythm entering your feet, energizing the muscles and organs as it flows upward. Allow your body to express the rhythm without impediment for at least fifteen more minutes. Be spontaneous.

When your dance is concluded, engage in two minutes of silent reflection. Be aware of the sensations in your body at rest. Monitor your breathing as it moves from a rapid to a relaxed rhythm. Thank God, the gods, or the universe for accepting your dance.

Walking Meditation

In the Soto school of Zen Buddhism, "just sitting" becomes the vehicle for enlightenment. By emulating the Buddha, the meditator observes the mind as it moves inward to a point of pure awareness. Another practice emphasizes attention in a similar situation, by focusing only on the body's natural movements. The idea of "action without motive" is applied to this style of meditation, so that the meditator is consciously engaged without a specific aim or motive. "Just doing" is the goal here. One form of this is *kinhin,* the Zen walking meditation.

ALERT

If you go to an unfamiliar religious or cultural site for meditation, be mindful of the guidelines and customs. For example, at mosques, churches, and temples, you may be asked to remove your shoes or cover your head. Show respect for other traditions, even if you may not agree with their dogma.

In the Zen walk, the erect posture of *zazen* ("sitting") is maintained; the only difference is that the lower half of the body is moving. The walker matches breath with each step and places mental focus solely on walking. He meditates on the body's movement and rhythm, not on the scenery. The walker moves silently in a clockwise direction. The Zen walk can be practiced wherever and whenever you are on foot. Whether on your morning constitutional or during a brief visit to the mall, mindful walking is a stimulating form of meditation.

Meditating in Nature

We all know how restorative nature can be. But nature as preventive medicine is now regarded as an important component in everyone's health regimen. Scientists at the Rollins School of Public Health at Emory University in Georgia suggest that a beautiful landscape may be a better remedy than medications in some instances. They explain that human beings possess a "habitat seeking" instinct, and the exercise of that best takes place in the natural environment. Four dimensions of the natural environment play into this instinct:

1. Contact with animals (wild in nature and pets)
2. Contact with plants (gardens, trees, houseplants)
3. Contact with wilderness (hiking, boating, camping)
4. Visual contact with landscapes (rolling hills, fields, mountains, forests)

The research noted that hospital patients healed more quickly when they were exposed to the natural environment. So it is no wonder that meditation in a natural environment increases the quotient for wellness and well-being considerably.

ESSENTIAL

If you want to meditate in a natural environment, look into visiting the accessible, large-scale natural environments close to you. Consider arboretums, botanical gardens, parks, meditation gardens, and memorial grounds.

Plan a meditative walk. Have a map or know the layout of the grounds so you won't lose track of your location. Bring appropriate foot and eyewear, layered clothing, and a water supply. Walk through the environment in a clockwise motion, beginning at the entrance, which we'll designate as six o'clock.

Stop for a meditative rest when you reach nine o'clock. Allow the sounds of the place to take precedence in your awareness. Move to twelve o'clock, and stop for another meditation. Allow the sights of the spot to take precedence. Continue to three o'clock, and pause for another reflective period. Allow the scents and textures of the location to take precedence.

Back at your starting point, take in the entire scene. Sounds, sights, and other sensations can now communicate the spirit of the place to you. You may want to return to one of the places you passed through for a concluding meditation.

Animal Meditation

Animal meditation is a wonderful way to relax and center oneself. Advocates of pet therapy affirm that the comforting presence of cats, dogs, birds, and fish in the home or office provide a calming influence. In some instances, attaching monitors to the owners confirms that blood pressure goes down, breathing is less labored, and physical pain is lessened.

Animals have the ability to ground us, because they bring the physical presence of nature directly into the environment. Closely tuned to the external world, animals hear the sounds we miss, and see the subtleties around them that we dismiss.

QUOTE

"If you wish to escape from suffering and fear, practice wisdom and compassion."
—Anatole France (1844–1924), French Nobel Prize winner for Literature, 1921

If you want to practice animal meditation, spend the same amount of time at the same time of day with your pet, even if it's five or ten minutes. The awareness of time in animals is remarkably high. Communicate in non-verbal ways. Gazing into the eyes, stroking, smiling, and gesturing are messages well understood by animals.

If you have problems, communicate them to your pet. They have a vast capacity for understanding and patience that you can access. If your pet is having problems, especially of a health nature, communicate your concern and love. They always acknowledge affection.

Wild animals can also spark meditative insights. Go into a wilderness area or park with an open, questioning frame of mind. You may want to work on some particular problem, but put it on hold for a while and allow the setting to speak to you. Find a place to sit down quietly for a while. You need not go out of your way to find animals: simply sit and listen. Animals live all around us and share our world. You need not see an exotic animal: a squirrel or a robin will do. Allow the experience of that animal to draw you away for a time. Enter its world for a while as you watch it feeding or playing or building a nest. You may take the time to jot down a few notes or make a sketch as an aid to attention. More often than not, you will emerge from the experience with a lighter frame of mind, often with an answer to that nagging problem. Take a minute or two to mentally say thanks to the other beings with whom we share our world and go through the day with an awareness of our interconnections with other species.

Everyday Moving Meditations

You may think that meditation in some places and environments is difficult, if not impossible. For instance, during the holidays you may often find yourself waiting in line at the post office or stuffed in a crowded room at a charity event. With nothing to do but wait, restlessness can easily set in. And there's nothing more irritating than waiting around with the person nearest you fidgeting nervously while another is rattling coins or keys in his pocket. Your inner voice may be crying, "Get me out of here!"

Instead, focus on a peaceful scene around you. It may be depicted in a painting on the wall or outside through a window. A sleeping baby in someone's arms or a patient, elderly person waiting nearby can provide the visual support that says to you, "Everything is moving in the right rhythm, and so am I."

But you have much more to do besides waiting in lines. The daily grind asks much of the inner resources, and meditation can support you along the way.

A Commuter's Meditation

You may experience the whole spectrum of negative emotions if you have to commute to work every day. Frustration, exasperation, rage—all result in stress. By the time you get to work, you are probably frazzled, and the coffee isn't going to help. What can you do while driving that will get you to work in a better frame of mind?

Focus on relaxing your body. Pay attention to what your mind is thinking about. Be sure to maintain a balance of both body and mind.

When you're commuting, noises are distracting but some can't be avoided. Choose uplifting music on the radio with minimal talk. Eliminate stressful news updates or traffic reports. Don't tap your fingers, feet, or hands, and avoid honking your car horn. Visually focus on careful driving.

ALERT

Don't race other cars to the stoplight; you will only gain a few seconds. Avoid critiquing other drivers. Acting like a trapped animal is useless. Just release and accept the situation.

In the meantime, nurture yourself. Stretch and relax your hands, one at a time. To de-stress, lift your shoulders up to your ears, release. Practice mantras; use tones for calming.

A Dieting Meditation

Many experts in diet and nutrition would probably agree that the problem of being overweight is not eating; it's the thought patterns of the person. Attitude—your view of yourself and food, how others see you, and how all those elements blend—is one dimension. Feeling—how food makes you feel in relation to what you can't feel (love, acceptance)—is another dimension. The last consideration is really the food itself, because that is more a side issue than the rest. As long as we can choose our food, we can choose a diet that is appropriate. But life is more than that. The complex of thinking and feeling takes the larger share.

Meditation for breaking bad habits and establishing good ones can include the basics that nearly all approaches use. Proper breathing, posture,

quiet time, reflection, and the development of openness to self are important. You can reverse bad habits by observing the passage of thoughts attentively. Think about whether there are some thoughts that lead to the desire
for food and comfort. Observe the passage of feelings and sensations as
well. Do some of them suggest emptiness or hunger?

Make no judgments about the cause or the blame. Make no resolutions.
Simply observe and make note of your observations.

Carry these observations into your daily life as much as possible. Notice
if some events, such as speaking with coworkers at your job or discussing a
problem with your partner, bring up the thoughts, feelings, and sensations
you noted in meditation. The objective is to become more familiar with the
situations that trigger the condition of eating to replace or compensate for
feelings. Observation leads to correction. Dr. Dean Ornish, the cardiovascular physician whose breakthrough program on reversing heart disease
utilizes meditation, has a suggestion called mindful tasting. Knowing that
chocolate, for example, may be off-limits in your diet doesn't mean you have
to do without it forever. Instead, try an exercise in mindful tasting.

At your meditation oasis, bring yourself to relaxation physically and mentally. Unwrap a modest amount of chocolate. A small bonbon of high quality
is a good choice. Place the chocolate in your mouth. Don't chew; don't ingest
it immediately. Allow the chocolate to melt slowly in your mouth. Hold it on
your tongue for as long as possible, savoring the taste and texture. Absorb
the chocolate essence into your being. Become the spirit of chocolate. In this
way, you don't deprive yourself of a food you love, and yet you don't overeat.

Meditation for a Test

Learning is potentially stressful. Besides understanding new material
and organizing it in ways you can recall, there is always competition and the
high expectations that go along with it. Altogether, these things do little to
inspire confidence when you are faced with turning points like taking a test.

Don't cram before a test. Take new material in small stages, spend
enough time until you understand it, and rest before going on to the next
stage. Meditate at least twenty minutes before studying. Regulate your breath
and posture; bring calm to your mind. Don't think about the test, and avoid
seeing yourself in the test environment. The only thought you can entertain
is the result of the test and what it means to you.

Always get enough rest before a test. Be sure to meditate before going to the test site. You want to arrive calm, relaxed, and confident.

ALERT

Don't throttle your thinking by trying to recall all you studied. If you studied well, it will reflect perfectly through a transparent mind. Seek that transparency.

Group Meditation and Releasing Emotions

How is it possible to be meditative if you are dealing with a group of people? Pop psychology gives plenty of lip service to forgiveness, releasing anger, bitterness, and dealing with pain and conflict with others. But there are few approaches that can be applied to every situation, and even fewer that deal with groups. Families, groups of workers, classes of students, clubs, and organizations—all of these units generate problems.

Once again, the Hawaiian culture provides a tradition that psychologists and social scientists admire. The ritual of *Ho'o ponopono* (ho-oh-po-no-po-no) means "to bring about order." This ritual is enacted because the culture believes in harmony, the key to health. Harmony doesn't just involve the individual. In this case, it includes the spiritual powers, fellow human beings, nature, and one's own being.

Ho'o ponopono is a group meditation, a spiritual work to mend interrelationships. A fivefold process is used to return harmony to the group, which takes meditative action at each stage. The group gathers and begins with group prayer. Everyone is reminded that a greater power is present that will be involved in the resolution of the problem.

The problem is stated. Each person in the group speaks of it and each person responds to what has been spoken. Each person exercises mindfulness. The group peels away the problem, seeking the fundamental reasons, feelings, and motivations. The members enter into reflective thought to discover any entanglements. The feelings and thoughts affected by the problem are brought out into the open. Insights are obtained. Each member of the group comes forward to resolve their involvement in the problem. Compassion is engaged. Then the group shares a meal to allow peace to settle and offers a prayer of solidarity. No member of the group will ever revisit the problem again, and so harmony is established.

The Tapestry of Life

In bygone days, things like weaving cloth and making furniture were necessary tasks of everyday life. At the same time, they were meditative experiences, like other daily chores. Time moved slowly; attention was focused on the work at hand. Such jobs were reduced to the simple exchange of physical energy with nature, enabling the mind to become clear. And without the distractions of television, industry, and traffic, the mind had no need to "tune out" the sounds of life. We admire people who maintain the simple calm of attending to the tasks of living, without regard to past concerns or future speculation.

There are many ways these same attitudes can be cultivated. Outside work or domestic tasks can become a vehicle for meditative experience. They can also be a test of your practice in focusing, calming, and mindfulness. Here are some physical activities that promote the meditative experience:

- Beadwork
- Carpentry
- Ceramics
- Cooking
- Doll making
- Painting
- Polishing
- Quilting
- Restoring
- Sewing
- Sketching
- Woodcarving

Mindful attention to these tasks, which engage the imagination, can lead to *noesis* ("creative insight"). Like art therapy, the thinking process is calmed in a way that joins physical activity with creative energy. Through these activities, opportunities arise for self-awareness, understanding, and healing.

CHAPTER 20

Coming Full Circle

Centuries of development and experiment have gone into meditation, and it's still not a static practice. Even science has ventured into the arena with laboratory tests and studies to discover why it appears to offer so much. But there is no standard way to meditate, and no test that can tell you what the best style of meditation is for your life.

Insight Meditation

One of the more widespread secular meditation techniques in the West is derived from a traditional Buddhist approach. Insight meditation is based on *samatha vipassana* (vippa-SA-na), a practice that seeks the development of calm and insight. Derived from the meditation approach of the Theravada school of Buddhism, it is regarded as the method by which the Buddha attained enlightenment. However, the spiritual tradition is not the focal point of this practice. Instead, this technique seeks to apply meditative experience to everyday life, and in this process the meditator's spiritual nature is developed.

According to the source teachings, the Buddha taught three essential guides to meditation. *Samatha* is the exercise of attention by calming the mind. *Vipassana* is the experience of insight. *Metta* is the development of "lovingkindness."

These guiding stages are not reached sequentially or according to a prescribed plan. They are experienced with respect to each person's experience. The three stages are really three dimensions that you can enter in a single meditation session. You may not feel as though you've worked through all three in any given session, or you may focus on one dimension for an extended period. Remember: It's based on your experience.

When you begin meditation, your attention may drift as a result of outside and inside interruptions. Of the latter, thoughts are the most persistent. But you don't have to push thoughts away, you can look at them as they appear in sequence and allow them to pass.

Begin insight meditation in the same manner as all the other traditions. You may prepare your space, do some preliminary reading or exercises, or just sit quietly to relax and release. Your breathing should be even and your posture upright.

Developing Samatha: Attention

In the first dimension, you work to sustain your attention on the present. Don't think of it as concentration, which implies forcing a frame of mind that you want to avoid. Gently bring your attention forward, to the here and now. Use breathwork, gentle exercise, and calm.

Developing Vipassana: Insight

In the second dimension, you reach a reflective condition. Your mind is transparent; it is only reflecting what is being seen, heard, and felt. The chatter is gone; the images are quiet. Now insight becomes possible.

When insight comes, it is marvelous. In most cases, you become aware of something that is new, but at the same time you knew it all along. Knowing and not knowing converge.

FACT

Jack Kornfield, PhD, joined the Peace Corps in 1967 and was assigned to Thailand, where he met a Buddhist teacher and studied meditation. Eventually, he became a monk and lived in Southeast Asia until 1972. He began to teach *vipassana* meditation, cofounding the Insight Meditation Society in Massachusetts. He now teaches insight meditation at a facility he founded, the Spirit Rock Center, near San Francisco.

If insight doesn't come, it doesn't matter, because you are in the stage of "meditation of being." You have entered a state of complete awareness with the immediate present; the inner and outer realities are one.

Developing Metta: Lovingkindness

In the third dimension, you are open to the inner and outer reality. The harmony of this state, where true oneness with life is achieved, opens the door to lovingkindness. The words loving and kindness are joined to indicate the attitude of all enlightened beings—Jesus, Buddha, Muhammad—and all the nameless ones who have gone before you. It is the acceptance of self and the world. It is the awakening of compassion.

How do you work toward this? Be soft. Meditation teachers say that while you are meditating, your heart should be soft and your belly should be soft. Overall, you should be relaxed, released, and open. In the process, you gain insight into how tough, rigid, and armored we become throughout the day. You notice how certain words and thoughts cause you to tense your muscles. You see how hard the body tries to deal with the assaults of daily life. In discovering these things, you also discover ways to ease those tensions and have lovingkindness toward yourself.

A Prayer for Lovingkindness

May every creature abound in well-being and peace.
May every living being, weak or strong, the long and the small,
The short and the medium-sized, the mean and the great,
May every living being seen or unseen,
Those dwelling far off, those nearby,
Those already born, those waiting to be born,
May all attain inward peace.
Let no one deceive another, let no one despise another in any situation.
Let no one, from antipathy or hatred, wish evil to anyone at all.
Just as a mother, with her own life protects her only son from hurt,
So within yourself foster a limitless concern for every creature.
Display a heart of boundless love for all the world,
In all its height and depth and broad extent.
Love unrestrained, without hate or enmity.
Then as you stand or walk, sit or lie, until overcome by drowsiness,
Devote your mind entirely to this, it is known as living here life divine.

Mindfulness Meditation

One of the aims of insight meditation is to understand the nature of the mind and become familiar with its workings. An important technique is the use of mindfulness throughout the meditation practice; that is, focused and sustained attention to what you are doing at the moment.

As simple as this sounds, mindfulness is not easily achieved. To start, one must be fully aware, and herein lies the challenge. Awareness comes in varying degrees, starting from babyhood through adolescence and adulthood, and into middle age and senescence. The engagement of the mind, feelings, and senses and energy levels are continually transforming. Even during a single day, awareness is minimal while sleeping and continually shifting while awake.

Being Mindful

Mindfulness is not confined to meditation. After developing this faculty as much as possible, you carry the awareness with you. It's applied to everything you do, from eating and working to learning and relaxing.

The experiences in each day, from the insignificant to the momentous, become rich and vibrant when you meet them with mindfulness. For most, it's not possible to engage mindfulness at each moment. But the practice is rewarding, and there will come a time when it becomes the way you live your life.

To live mindfully, narrow your attention to the task at hand. Avoid flying from one thought to another, or from thinking to feeling. All senses should be intent on what you are doing. Train the mind to be transparent, to reflect what is in the moment. This eliminates speculation (future) and prejudice (past).

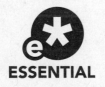

ESSENTIAL

Accepting yourself and others is a way to avoid stress and fear. Be kind and exercise patience, most of all to and with yourself. Observe the sensations and thoughts that enter your consciousness. Allow them to pass through.

Apply what you discover in this process to real life. Having breakthroughs in understanding is wonderful, but they are useless until put into action.

A Mindful Exercise

An exercise in mindfulness meditation usually starts by focusing on the physical body and then moving to the mind.

Start by using a technique of "scanning" or "sweeping" the body from bottom to top. Start with the feet; move up in sequence to the calves, thighs, torso, arms, neck, and head.

Move your focus slowly. With eyes closed, train your attention on each section of your body. Note the sensations of heat and cold, the air on your skin, the texture of the muscles, any stiffness, any pulsing sensations. Give yourself ten minutes for this.

When you have finished with your head, move your attention to breathing. Note its evenness and rhythm. Give yourself five minutes for this.

Now relax your attention and observe your thoughts. If thinking interferes with observing, go back to scanning your body.

A Mindfulness Meditation Luminary

John Kabat-Zinn has investigated and taught mindfulness meditation in a therapeutic setting since 1979. As founder of the Stress Reduction Clinic at the University of Massachusetts Memorial Medical Center, Kabat-Zinn was featured on the acclaimed public-television series *Healing and the Mind*, hosted by Bill Moyers. Kabat-Zinn took the theme of experiencing life's ebb and flow—the "full catastrophe" described by Zorba the Greek—as a metaphor for the engaged mind. Kabat-Zinn espouses awareness and acceptance as the keys to experiencing life fully, along with the development of grace and humor. He also trains meditation teachers in an eight-week program for developing healthy attitudes and behaviors.

Making Peace with Yourself

Self-acceptance is one of the goals in mindfulness meditation. When you observe the thoughts that pass through your mind, you should observe your reactions to them as well. What you may not expect is the criticism that you often level at yourself—for example, thinking "wrong" versus "right" thoughts about yourself or others, your action or lack of action in recalled situations. These patterns of thinking come from conditioning and past experience, and they are of no use in growing and understanding.

Not judging yourself is difficult enough. But when the criticism and high expectations diminish, you need to nourish yourself. Meditation is a way of addressing that, but insights may come for opening your heart to the fullness of life you seek.

Meditation for Survival

Is lovingkindness wired into the brain? University of Virginia psychologist Jonathan Haidt believes it is. Every emotion has a "constellation" of physical symptoms—a measurable reaction in the body brought on by feelings. For example, anger will cause flushed skin, narrowing of the eyes, and acceleration of the heartbeat. In fact, researchers have identified six emotions that have significant effects on the body: anger, fear, disgust, happiness, sadness, and surprise. But Haidt proposes that there is a seventh emotion, and he calls it "elevation."

QUOTE

"Meditation is giving yourself permission to be free."

—Anonymous

Seeing acts of charity and kindness affects many people with sensations of expansion, tears, and chills. Haidt and his colleagues propose that those feelings can inspire and affect moral behavior, so they conducted a study on subjects who watched a documentary about Mother Teresa. Afterward, viewers reported wanting to participate in similar activities, such as volunteering.

Psychologists point out that all of our feelings arise from eons of conditioning for survival. If the emotion of elevation is part of this, then meditation for developing lovingkindness stands to be one of our survival tools.

Choiceless Meditation

One of the great figures in the twentieth-century consciousness movement was Jeddu Krishnamurti, a spiritual teacher and meditation educator. Born in India in 1895 to a poor family, he was "discovered" at the age of ten by C. W. Leadbeater, a controversial figure in the early Theosophical Society. According to Leadbeater's clairvoyant perception of the young Hindu, he was destined to become a great leader, the next avatar or reincarnation of the world teacher.

Krishnamurti struggled with the burden of preparing to be the world teacher while reaching maturity. He displayed unusual sensitivity to the problems of individuals and society, a quality he would possess throughout his life. But at the age of twenty-nine, he dissolved the large following that had gathered around him and declared that he would not play the role he had been assigned. In an earth-shattering statement, he told his disciples, "Truth is a pathless land. Man cannot come to it through any organization, through any creed, through any dogma, priest or ritual, not through any philosophic knowledge or psychological technique." (Lutyens, Mary, *Krishnamurti—The Years of Awakening.* [New York: Avon Books, 1991]) He spent the rest of his life showing others the way to live that statement until he passed away in 1986.

The foundation Krishnamurti established to consolidate and spread his wisdom teaches a meditative process in the tradition of Raja Yoga. He used the term "choiceless awareness" to describe his approach, and it has become a well-regarded style of meditation. It is akin to the mindfulness of Buddhist *vipassana,* where only focus and attentiveness are sought. One stays in the moment, without expectation or goals. There is no thinking, feeling, or recollection.

This state is said to attract energy from without. In the process, awareness becomes even more elevated. And so it continues, until the observer and the observed become a unity.

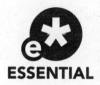

ESSENTIAL

> If you want to try guided meditation, start by being calm and relaxed, at complete rest on the outside and the inside. Take a deep breath, exhaling peacefully. Closing your eyes, feel warmth surrounding you like a cocoon. It is protective and secure, assuring you that your rest will not be disturbed.

Guided Meditation and Scripts

Creative visualization is a process that engages your imagination. You can guide it to produce a result, or allow it to take place spontaneously, as in a daydream. You can produce a result by starting with some type of input and visualizing a finished object. For example, an architect might be given a construction budget, a designated space, and some style ideas. The architect's imagination would do the rest. Her creative visualization would bring a finished project into being.

Guided meditation usually follows a script that is unfamiliar to the meditator, but not always. The guide may be your own voice (prerecorded) or a meditation coach or teacher, live or recorded. The script's purpose is to place you in a meditative state, but it should have a specific goal that both you and the guide fully understand and agree on. Guided meditation can be used as an orientation tool rather than your sole approach to meditation. When it is being guided, your imagination can only be extended so far. After that, the experience of true reality cannot be "imagined," it can only be experienced.

Meditation or Hypnosis?

In Yoga, hypnosis is called *vasikaranam,* a state akin to mind control. It's not regarded very highly, because meditation in this tradition is the individual's complete mastery of the mental functions. To place that in someone else's hands is wrong, according to this system.

FACT

Meditation and hypnosis have some things in common. They can both address thought patterns that are destructive to health and well-being, and they can both increase your awareness of conditions that are ordinarily overlooked. One major difference, however, is that meditation seeks to awaken all dimensions of your mind and perceptions, while hypnosis hones in on a specific area of your thinking and feeling functions.

On the other hand, hypnosis has a number of valuable therapeutic attributes. It is used to successfully treat obesity, addiction, phobias, and pain. In the hands of a trained, clinical hypnotist, a person can benefit tremendously from the technique.

Contrary to the way it is portrayed in movies and sideshows, you are not "asleep" while you are hypnotized. In fact, your awareness of everything around you is rather acute. However, it is in command of the hypnotist. If you have a very strong sense of individuality, you will make a difficult subject. This is what distinguishes meditation from hypnosis. Your willingness to surrender to the hypnotist is essential for this method to work.

You can accomplish the same things through meditation that you would treat with hypnosis. It will take longer, naturally, even if you are working with a meditation coach. However, the results will last longer. Hypnosis can get to the source of a problem or issue quickly, but it requires continued reinforcement for it to work over a long period. Follow-up counseling and exercises, which often include meditation, are usually recommended in the course of hypnotic therapy.

Transcendental Meditation

When the Beatles went off to Bangor, Wales, in 1967 to sit at the feet of a meditation teacher, they were satirized by some and admired by others. Taking such an extended break away from "civilization" at the time was amazing. What could the odd, mystical-looking little guru possibly have to offer them that success didn't?

FACT

Deepak Chopra, a trained endocrinologist who also practices Ayurveda, the Hindu stream of metaphysical medicine, studied under Maharishi Mahesh Yogi.

Since then, the simple teachings of Maharishi Mahesh Yogi have transformed the realm of mind-body science and contributed largely to the new "meditation culture" of the Western world. The Maharishi's technique, called transcendental meditation (TM), is now taught at centers, businesses, and in private homes around the world. It teaches the basic methods for mental relaxation through recitation of a personal mantra. These methods cannot be learned by reading books or listening to tapes; they must be received through live instruction. A substantial fee is charged for the instruction, and additional training at extra expense is often encouraged.

One of the important aims of transcendental meditation is deep rest. It is regarded as the optimum remedy to the stresses of modern life, and has been confirmed by plenty of scientific research funded by the organization. In fact, most of the existing medical studies that confirm the value of meditation have been derived using meditators employing the TM technique.

What's Your Type?

In the early 1980s, psychologists began to associate personality traits with certain health problems. This set one of the first benchmarks in body-mind medicine, and clinicians continue to look at the phenomenon of illness as more engaged with states of mind than previously believed. First, type A and type B personalities were established, and behavioral profiles of these personality types were associated with common diseases in industrial societies.

Type A Personality

Type A personality behaviors are associated with coronary heart disease and stroke. These traits include aggression, leading to hostility toward others; impatience, or a sense of urgency; achievement orientation, leading to excessive competitiveness; and insecurity, which leads to "overstriving."

Meditation can be particularly valuable in this situation. Modern culture promotes—and at times rewards and elevates—the type A personality. But the health risks this brings far outweigh those rewards. Even if an individual remains in this typology throughout life, at least in meditation he can cultivate a type B attitude.

Type B Personality

The type B personality is more responsive to relaxing activities. But according to research, type B personalities make up only about 10 percent of the U.S. population. A type B usually follows his own rhythm in time and work habits, is patient and willing to wait, is comfortable with his current goals, and rarely exhibits hostility or insecurity.

Meditation and Healing

In medicine, the term psychosomatic refers to illness that arises from both mental and physical causes. It does not mean that an illness is "all in the mind." Rather, it describes conditions of the body that can be treated through the mind. Some physicians believe about 90 percent of all illnesses (including accidents) are psychosomatic.

One technique used to accelerate the healing processes meditatively is the use of creative visualization. This is a way of engaging the mind with the illness, and using it to connect with and counter the organic processes that have brought about the condition.

Holistic healers have an interesting way of looking at illness. For every crisis, they say, there is an opportunity. That event is not only an opportunity for healing, but a possibility for learning important lessons that will lead to a far more meaningful life.

In this vein, researchers have discovered that at the crisis stage of an illness, the consciousness of the patient is particularly acute. Scientists are unsure whether this state is brought on by fever, shock, fear, or the profound acceptance of mortality. Whatever the reason, the mind becomes unusually sharp and multidimensional (enabling the recall of forgotten events with clarity, for example), which presents an opportunity for bridging the separation between body and mind, and engaging the two in a reversal of the condition.

Through meditative work, patients in critical condition or with life-threatening illnesses have reversed their illnesses or at least diminished the painful symptoms. If an organ is affected, creative visualization is employed to see it mending. If a disease has attacked the body, the same method is used to expel the virus or cancer. And if a degenerative condition is at work, visualizations combined with breathwork and Yogic body vitalizations are engaged to subvert the decline.

In essence, healing meditation addresses the body to mend via the visualization mechanism. Supportive techniques from Yoga bodywork and Buddhist mental exercises are also incorporated. And prayer cannot be discounted as a powerful tool in becoming whole. Nearly every meditation tradition has a niche for healing meditation, and they should be explored fully if you have a health problem that you want to work through.

Of course, healthful living is the ultimate remedy. But that is a path that includes meditation, so you might as well begin now.

What the Traditions Teach

The practice of meditation is beneficial only when it is incorporated into the routine of everyday life. Meditation must be continuous and spontaneous to be effective, not an occasional "event" that removes us from reality. In fact, meditation is the experience of true reality, and for that reason it should be made a part of each day.

Each meditation tradition has something unique to offer. You may not adopt a single tradition that agrees with your personality and experience. But you may find something in each that can contribute to your personal growth. Here are some of those themes:

Tradition	Teaching
Buddhism	Compassion
Christianity	Devotion
Hatha Yoga	Harmony
Insight	Mindfulness
Kabbalism	Vision
Raja Yoga	Focus
Ritual	Sacredness
Shamanism	Kinship
Sufism	Joy
Tantra Yoga	Interrelationship
Taoism	Balance
Zen	Stillness

CHAPTER 21

Mind and Beyond

You can put meditation to use right away in your own life, whether you're having trouble sleeping or you want a better way to relate to your friends and family. But meditation does occasionally present some side effects that you will need to work through. Here are some final tips you need to know before you dive into the world of meditation.

Meditation and Sleep

In any given year, at least half of the American population will have difficulty falling asleep. Even worse, sleep researchers have found that up to one-third of us aren't getting enough sleep. Insomnia is caused by many factors; some may arise from medical and environmental conditions. But the most common causes are tension, anxiety, and depression.

Drug intervention is the most common approach to dealing with insomnia, but both doctors and patients know that this is just a temporary measure. Drugs will induce sleep, but they interfere with the process of rapid eye movement (REM), which is necessary for rejuvenating sleep. In this process, the brain reaches the theta state (sleep transition), where dream activity occurs.

Causes of Insomnia

In many cases, insomnia stems from an anxiety-related disorder. Any of the following forms of emotional turbulence can lead to anxiety-related sleep problems:

- **Change:** Environmental, climatic, seasonal
- **Emotional stimulation:** Excitement from meaningful events
- **Fear:** Recent trauma, anticipation of unwanted conditions
- **Frustration:** Emotional and sexual
- **Health concerns:** Recent illness, glandular changes, pain
- **Mental stimulation:** Extended periods of learning, television viewing
- **Physical stimulation:** Diet, drugs, alcohol, caffeine
- **Worry:** Money, health, relationships

Rare is the person who has not experienced a few of these conditions. Meditation alone may not address all of them, but when used in combination with other natural treatments, it can accelerate the return to well-being. While more work still needs to be done in this area, several studies have shown a connection between meditation and improved sleep quality.

Of course, the inverse is also true: a good night's sleep leads to a more attentive meditation session. Almost everyone has taken a short nap while meditating, and sometimes sleep is what the body most needs. But meditation should be about more than sleep, so try to maintain good sleeping habits to support your meditation practice. The Himalayan Academy recommends practicing meditation during the hours before dawn (yes, that early!) five days a week, taking the weekend mornings to rest and recuperate. The most important thing, for both sleep and meditation, is to establish regular patterns. Then you will be working with your body's rhythms instead of against them.

A Sleep Meditation

Getting established in a regular meditation practice will encourage regular, deeper sleep. We recommend two sessions per day, one in the morning and one in the evening, lasting twenty minutes each (see track one on the CD that accompanies this book). That said, you may find yourself lying awake at night, not knowing what to do in order to get to sleep. The following brief meditation will help.

It's easier to fall asleep when your body is relaxed. Naturally, this is difficult to achieve when you are worried and tense. But simple muscle-toning exercises can help.

Pranayama exercises (conscious breathing) should accompany a sleep meditation because the assistance they render is invaluable. Good oxygenation will induce a relaxed state and encourage yawning—always a good sign.

FACT

Sleep scientists at Oxford University recently reported that instructing patients to divert their thoughts with other thoughts (such as counting sheep) fails to induce sleep. However, the researchers found that visualizing a peaceful, calm scene had their subjects dozing off more quickly than any other. Meditation, anyone?

Lie on your back, hands on stomach, legs extended, eyes half closed. Avoid curling your body in a ball or lying on your side. Gradually focus on your body, from the feet up. Focus your attention only on your bodywork. Starting with the feet, turn them in and curl your toes downward, as tightly as possible. As you do this, inhale. Release slowly while exhaling. Move to your calves, turn them inward and tighten the muscles while inhaling. Release slowly while exhaling. Now focus on your thighs, tightening the muscles while inhaling. Release slowly while exhaling. Move your attention to the torso. As you inhale, allow your stomach to expand fully. Slowly exhale. Tensing, release your hands while inhaling and exhaling. Do the same with your arms and hands, while raising your shoulders upward toward your ears. Inhale; exhale while tensing and releasing. Tense your head by raising your chin upward as far as possible while inhaling. Slowly release it downward while exhaling. Avoid twisting your neck to the right or left. Perform three conscious breaths while wriggling your fingers and toes.

Dream Meditation

What do dreams have in common with meditation? For starters, they are methods by which we may understand deeper levels of ourselves. Feelings, impressions, memories, and intuition all form a part of our life perception. But we often don't pay enough attention to them. By recording and studying our dreams, we can discover strengths we overlook, and even resolve problems we once thought were insurmountable. These are also processes by which we can develop more awareness, which is one of the primary goals of meditation.

FACT

Ancient cultures saw certain dreams as omens, pictures of future events in symbolic form. These dreams occur quite often, and there are many explanations for it. The best one is that by paying attention to your dreams, you are tapping into your own timeless dimension.

The objective of dream meditation is to exercise attention and mindfulness while in the dream state, just as in the meditative state. At the same time, you are making the unconscious dimension accessible. This makes it easier to "break through" everyday thoughts and feelings and reach the deeper stillness of meditation.

Dream meditation is very simple, but it requires dedication: you will need to practice it consistently. Once you decide to pursue it, incorporate it in your daily regimen. There are few tools, just a journal for recording your dreams and a lamp near your sleeping area. You may awaken early and want to write down a dream immediately.

Record your dreams on awaking. Never do it later; the details will be lost or even forgotten. Take the time to write down the dream from beginning to end. If you do not recall a dream when you wake up, open the journal and record the date with "no dream." Remember: The habit you are establishing is as important as the dream content itself.

Read your dream journal at your meditation oasis. If you aren't able to do this, read the journal before you retire in your sleeping area. After reading the dream, close your eyes and place yourself in the dream once more. Pay attention to the details of the environment, the persons with you, the words said, and the actions performed. Open your eyes and reread the recorded dream. Are there details your meditation revealed that are not recorded? If so, add them as an "afterword."

After comparing what you read with what you recalled, reflect on the meaning. You will discover unopened messages as you go through the process of recording, reading, recalling, and reflecting.

Dreams are like unopened letters. They contain important messages, but we have to devote the time to reading them and reflecting on their meaning. Make note of details in your dreams. Clothing, words, and scenery are clues to meaning because the unconscious communicates in symbols. Dreams will reveal patterns. They may appear in the form of consistent symbols, scenarios, or feelings. It's important to look at and reflect on these patterns.

Draw out floor plans and patterns that you see in dreams. Many neurologists ask this of patients, to determine how they understand space in relation to themselves.

Daydreaming

One of the first problems encountered in meditation is the tendency to daydream ("waking dream"). Daydreaming is the result of the mind's active need for stimulation while attempting repose. For example, you may be entering a meditation session with the intention of clearing your mind of the day's concerns. As you try to accomplish this, an image of a sailboat appears in your mind. You may dismiss it, but the sailboat returns and this time you are at the helm. Giving into the scene, you are on the sailboat on a calm ocean. Friends appear on deck, and you are celebrating a birthday. Your longed-for gift of a telescope is presented, and you set it up immediately to look at the stars.

Research in biofeedback shows that subjects who are daydreaming reflect alpha brain wave activity, a relaxed state. In this condition, we are fulfilling unrealized wishes, escaping the stresses of a harsh reality, and living vicariously in situations not yet possible.

The one dimension employed in daydream that distinguishes the process from true meditation is the imagination. Using words, pictures, sounds, and other sense phenomena can easily stimulate the imagination, and from there the mental "drama" takes off.

Pioneering space scientist Robert Goddard supposedly developed his design for rocket-powered space vehicles while daydreaming. One day as he was spending time high in a cherry tree at his New England home, he daydreamed about going to Mars. That and similar daydreams led him to study astronomy, physics, and aeronautics. Goddard's daydreams eventually became reality, and his experiences in this realm inspired a valuable contribution to future science.

ESSENTIAL

Recall a place that holds positive memories for you. It may be a childhood hideout, a vacation getaway, or a country you've visited. Recall as many details as possible: the weather, environmental features, the architecture. Choose a familiar spot in this scenario, and place yourself in it, as you are now. See what happens.

Such experiences are similar to techniques used in meditation. Sense phenomena can be used as "launching points" for attaining separation from ordinary mental activities. But at this juncture an important decision must be made. Will the mind now journey in a designated direction, or will it journey to a destination of its own choosing? Here lies the difference between meditation (designated direction) and daydream (destination without choice).

Wishing

Wishing is akin to daydream activity, but is different from "wishful thinking," which is self-deception. Wishful thinking places you in a situation that has no relation to the past or present reality. True wishing engages both imagination and memory in anticipation of a specific goal. In this case, you place yourself in a situation that proceeds from the present to a future reality. It's similar to seeing a movie in fast-forward.

Some meditation techniques use precisely this mechanism, calling it by other names, such as creative visualization or conscious imagining. But the premise is the same, using your conscious faculties to shape future possibilities based on what is important to you in the present. Is this practical?

Visualizing goals is practical and in most cases, necessary. Since you are the person who is most aware of your strengths and weaknesses, realizing a wish is going to become more likely once you have considered all possible avenues.

Here's an approach to productive wishing: Consider one wish only. Clarify it mentally, using a minimal number of words. For example, "I wish to go to Bali when I get my raise at work" is not a single goal with minimal considerations. Rather, "I wish to be in Bali" is a personal, meaningful goal that is independent of qualifications.

Immerse yourself in the experience of the wish. In this case, being in Bali could get some help from travel brochures and ambient music so you can see the sights and hear the sounds of this locale. The goal is to become as familiar as possible with the elements of the wish.

See yourself in the locale, performing the actions that reflect your wish. Walk on the beach; hike up a rain-forest mountain. Pan into the scene closely, using the details you've learned. Pan out of the locale, back to the present. Limit your visits to the wish place to once a day. This is a "transporting meditation," in which you transport your attention to another dimension where you can see the vista of an experience.

Potential Dangers

Can the practice of meditation bring problems? Are there dangers? These questions may seem absurd, but there are some aspects of the meditation experience that can present problems. The Yogic and Buddhist traditions speak of this quite matter-of-factly. They point out that working with the mind and emotions is a serious business, and some pitfalls may be encountered. That's why advanced techniques call for an experienced teacher to guide the practitioner through such events without difficulty.

Going Overboard

An early temptation in meditation practice is to launch into it with abandon, even neglecting other duties. The feelings of bliss that sometimes come with meditation can act as a lure. It can be tempting to think, "If a little bit is good, more must be better." Instead, settle into a daily routine of one morning and one evening session, and consider going on a monthly, day-long retreat. Anything more than this is likely to be counter-productive. Make sure to complete your daily duties even better than you did in the past: this will springboard your practice more than multi-hour meditation sessions.

Another important caution is to avoid extreme practices, at least in the beginning. You may run into books on fasting and other physical disciplines, but these should only be pursued under the supervision of a physician and with the guidance of a qualified spiritual leader. Beginners may run the risk of treating the body too harshly and ultimately create psychological problems instead of eliminating them.

Hearing Strange Sounds

With awareness tuned to a greater degree, sounds may become audible that have no identity or apparent origin. Some Zen practitioners have reported hearing thunderclaps, while students of Yoga may hear the sounds of rushing water or air. These may be the sounds of the eardrums adjusting to changes in pressure while performing breathing or Yoga exercises. Likewise, certain postures can cause the vertebrae or ankles to make cracking noises. With your hearing more acute in these situations, sounds are more distracting.

Feeling Physical Pain

You may encounter headaches, stomachaches, or back pain as you become still and more aware of your body. Go at a slower pace and relax your expectations of what you'll get from meditation practice. Don't strain. Remember that meditation is not a way to discipline or force yourself into "being good."

ALERT

Be mindful of any pain, and trace it to the source as much as you are able. Consult with your physician about what you've experienced and what you perceive as the cause.

Panic Attacks

As the awareness process develops, you may begin to feel that you are losing control. Remind yourself that you have made the decision to enter new territory and that you are always in charge. You can pause for a while or go forward, but avoid giving up because you think you have "failed." One important technique in handling panic is to surrender to the feeling and not fight it. That diminishes its power.

Hearing Voices

As the unconscious mind becomes more accessible through meditation, some of its contents may become conscious spontaneously. This can come in the form of previously forgotten conversations and the voices of persons past and present. Here is one of the more serious pitfalls that can lock a person into states of thinking that are unrealistic and hazardous. Speaking with the dead, contacting alien intelligences, and being guided by spiritual figures are part of the landscape of this phenomenon. They have not only become topics of serious discussion in the mind-body-spirit movement; they have become adversely exploited in the entertainment and marketing industries. Exercise caution here.

All meditation traditions warn of becoming drawn into "dependent" states of mind. These are stages of belief where the meditator becomes dependent on a "higher" influence for decisions and actions. As with everything that is encountered in the practice of self-awareness, these stages are inconsequential to the goal of enlightenment.

Countering Activities

Although some potential problems can occur in meditation, it is not a dangerous activity. It is natural, beneficial, and stands up to the test of time as a means of achieving self-knowledge. There are ways that you can ensure a positive practice throughout your exploration of this vital path, and you should consider them at times.

ALERT

As long as you are not in any physical pain or discomfort, allow the noises to pass into the distance and don't invite more by anticipating them. Maintain your meditation focus.

If you feel blocked (the perception that you are not accomplishing anything, not moving forward or inward), consider trying another style of meditation. If you are practicing Yoga *asanas* and breathing, move to a type of Zen stillness. Conversely, if you are engaged in deep meditative exercise, consider a walking or ritual meditative activity.

If you dread a meditation session (expecting too much effort or negative results), remember that you are not doing this to accomplish anything. Rather, you are just doing it "to be." Here, a form of devotional meditative activity may steer you to develop lovingkindness toward yourself.

If you can't seem to settle into meditation, you may be trying to do too much at once. For example, learning breathing, posture, mental stillness, and creative visualization while rearranging your meditation oasis may be scattering your focus. Instead, be attentive to just one thing at a time, and be patient.

Going deep into the mental stratosphere requires very small steps. If you get a scary feeling sometimes in meditation, take breaks within your sessions. Have tea, read an inspirational piece, take a vitalizing breath. Then return to the practice.

The Importance of Exercise and Diet

Try not to use meditation as an excuse to avoid other healthful practices: all of the standard health advice still holds, no matter how adept you become at entering altered states of consciousness. Adopting a vegetarian diet, for example, can be beneficial for meditators and nonmeditators alike. Vegetarians live longer on average, have fewer problems with weight gain, have lower rates of heart disease, and may be less susceptible to certain kinds of cancer. The benefits to your practice lie in maintaining a more harm-free lifestyle in keeping with the practice of meditation. Avoiding heavy, fatty foods and processed foods, including refined sugar, may help boost energy levels and eliminate negative emotions.

Meditation has some of the same benefits as physical exercise, but by no means should it be regarded as a substitute for exercise. An hour of exercise a day will maintain vibrant health and cut through obstacles at a much greater rate than meditation alone. Think of meditation as one tool in your wellness kit, as part of an overall package of ethical living, physical exercise, healthy diet, and recreational activities. Those who pursue meditation as part of this overall package will see much greater improvement in quality of life than those who rely on meditation alone. Meditators will also see more improvements in health than those who rely simply on exercise and diet.

Meditation Attitudes

As you progress in your meditation experience, new worlds of awareness and insight will open to you. This is especially valuable in creative work and it makes your everyday life meaningful and productive. You will find your attitude changing about some things; it will always be for the better. For example, you may understand the discomforts of others because you are more aware of their pain or difficulties. In turn, you will be more patient with yourself, sensing how your own discomforts should be addressed as well. Still, there are some attitudes to avoid; many of them stem from the habits of everyday life.

Meditation should never be used to influence others. The insights you receive through this practice should be put to practical use in your own life, not paraded as newfound revelations to friends. For example, if your friend asks you, "What do you think I should do about this relationship?," don't say, "Get rid of that person, it's the best thing you can do. I got that yesterday in meditation." Here, your meditation is being used to influence a decision that should have been made through the friend's meditation.

Meditation should never become an excuse to avoid responsibility. For example, if you have promised to run errands for the family and you put it off because of your busy schedule, who are you letting down? If your spouse says, "Didn't you say you could pick up my package at the post office?" and you reply, "Why can't you take care of that? It's time for my meditation," then you're using meditation in a negative way.

Meditation should never be used to promote yourself at the expense of others. This happens in an environment where competition and insecurity go unchecked, and neither is conducive to meditative wisdom.

FACT

Here's an example of promoting yourself at the expense of others: Your neighbor says, "I'm really getting a lot of insight from the gardening course at the nursery," and you reply, "I get so much more insight out of meditation these days. Who needs gardening?"

In many examples, there are opportunities for meditative action. We can counter attitudes that offset our commitment to a good practice. All it takes is the use of mindfulness when we deal with everyday situations. The first step is to pause in these situations and consider: What is the best way to demonstrate the qualities I'm seeking through meditation? For example, you could say to your friend, "If you meditate on your situation, you will surely discover what to do about this relationship." To your spouse, you could reply, "Don't worry, I'm learning how to be mindful of my promises."

Meditating on Yourself

You are the result of millions of repetitive thoughts and actions. You do not come into this world finished; you are always in the process of becoming something more and someone else. Within this stream of growth, there are also millions of choices you are making and will soon make that will affect what you are and will be.

Now is the time to pause and look at this process. You can initiate this with an exercise in self-inquiry. Write the following questions on separate pieces of paper, and reflect on each one in turn.

1. What am I now?
2. What should I be?
3. What do I want to be?
4. How can I be all of that?

After you have reviewed all the images and ideas that these questions present, pause once more. Put the questions away and then reflect on these words:

I am what I am now, and what I should be.
I am what I want to be.
I am the future within all time.
I live in the present and in the Infinite.
I exist in the center of the world of life.

Taking into account the many approaches to meditation practice over eons of time and among the countless cultures in this world, the goal remains the same. Through it, we come to an understanding that we are more than flesh and blood. We are gifted with mind, heart, and spirit. And all of us, no matter what our condition, are given the opportunity to explore those dimensions. Meditation is a way of unifying them, to become more than the sum of our parts.

APPENDIX A

Suggested Reading

Chapter 1

Moyers, Bill. *Healing and the Mind* (New York: Doubleday, 1993).

Ornish, Dean. *Dr. Dean Ornish's Program for Reversing Heart Disease* (New York: Ballantine Books, 1990).

Chapter 2

Alberts, Bruce, Dennis Bray, et al. *Essential Cell Biology*. 3rd Edition. (New York: Garland, 2010).

Jerath, Ravinder. *Pranayama: Converting Stress and Anxiety into Inner Joy*. (Bloomington, Indiana: AuthorHouse, 2010). Website with supplementary material: *http://149588.myauthorsite.com*

Kohn, Livia. *Meditation Works: In the Daoist, Buddhist, and Hindu Traditions*. (Magadalena, NM: Three Pines, 2008).

Shusterman, Richard. *Body Consciousness: A Philosophy of Mindfulness and Somaesthetics*. (Cambridge: Cambridge University Press, 2008).

Sugunasiri, Suwanda H. J. "The Whole Body, Not Heart, as 'Seat of Consciousness': The Buddha's View." *Philosophy East and West* 45, No. 3 (1995): 409–430.

Chapter 3

Chopra, Deepak. *Ageless Body, Timeless Mind* (New York: Crown Publishers, 1993).

Grof, Stanislav. *The Adventure of Self Discovery* (Albany: SUNY Press, 1988).

Chapter 4

Farhi, Donna. *The Breathing Book: Good Health and Vitality Through Essential Breath Work* (New York: Owl Books, 1996).

Miller, Elise Browning. *Life Is a Stretch: Easy Yoga, Anytime, Anywhere* (St. Paul, MN: Llewellyn Publications, 1999).

Chapter 5

Linn, Denise. *Sacred Space: Clearing and Enhancing the Energy of Your Home* (New York: Ballantine Books, 1995).

Chapter 6

Feuerstein, Georg. *Shambhala Encyclopedia of Yoga* (Boston: Shambhala Publications, 1997).

Chapter 7

Christensen, Alice. *The American Yoga Association's Beginner's Manual* (New York: Simon & Schuster Trade Paperbacks, 2002).

Pegrum, Juliet, and Ambikananda Saraswati. *Ashtanga Yoga: The Complete Mind and Body Workout* (New York: Sterling Publishing Co., 2001).

Chapter 8

Anodea, Judith. *Wheels of Life: A User's Guide to the Chakra System* (St. Paul, MN: Llewellyn Publications, 1987).

Yogananda, Paramahansa. *Autobiography of a Yogi* (Nevada City, CA: Crystal Clarity Publications, 1995).

Chapter 9

Chodron, Pema. *Places That Scare You: A Guide to Fearlessness in Difficult Times* (Boston: Shambhala Publications, 2001).

Das, Lama Surya. *Awakening the Buddhist Heart: Integrating Love, Meaning, and Connection into Every Part of Your Life* (New York: Broadway Books, 2001).

Kornfield, Jack. *A Still Forest Pool* (Wheaton, IL: Quest Books, 1985).

Snelling, John. *The Buddhist Handbook* (Rochester, VT: Inner Traditions International, 1991).

Chapter 10

Rahula, Walpola. *What the Buddha Taught* (New York: Grove Press, 1974).

Rinpoche, Sogyal. *The Tibetan Book of Living and Dying* (San Francisco: HarperSanFrancisco, 1992).

Trungpa, Chogyam. *Training the Mind and Cultivating Loving-Kindness* (Boston: Shambhala Publications, 1993).

Chapter 11

Chia, Mantak. *Awaken Healing Energy Through the Tao* (New York: Aurora Press, 1983).

Lao Tzu. *Tao Te Ching*. Translated by Jonathan Star (New York: Putnam Publishing Group, 2001).

Chapter 12

Fontana, David. *Discover Zen: A Practical Guide to Personal Serenity* (San Francisco: Chronicle Books, 2001).

Sluyter, Dean. *The Zen Commandments: Ten Suggestions for a Life of Inner Freedom* (New York: Putnam Publishing Group, 2001).

Thich Nhat Hanh. *Anger* (New York: Putnam Publishing Group, 2001).

Thorp, Gary. *Sweeping Changes: Discovering the Joy of Zen in Everyday Tasks* (New York: Broadway Books, 2001).

Chapter 13

Barks, Coleman, trans. *The Essential Rumi* (New York: Castle Books, 1997).

Guénon, René. *Fundamental Symbols: The Universal Language of Sacred Science* (Cambridge, UK: Quinta Essentia, 1995).

Chapter 14

Furlong, Monica, ed. *Women Pray: Voices Through the Ages, from Many Faiths, Cultures, and Traditions* (Woodstock, VT: SkyLight Paths, 2001).

Merton, Thomas. *New Seeds of Contemplation* (New York: W.W. Norton & Co., 1974).

Monk of the Eastern Church, A. *The Jesus Prayer.* Foreword by Kallistos Ware. (Crestwood, NY: St. Vladimir's Seminary Press, 1987).

St. Teresa of Ávila. *The Interior Castle* (New York: Doubleday, 1972).

Sand, Annette, ed., and R. M. French, trans. *The Way of a Pilgrim* (Pasadena, CA: Hope Publishing House, 1993).

Chapter 15

Jette, Christine. *Tarot for the Healing Heart* (St. Paul: Llewellyn Publications, 2001).

Rosenthal, Norman. *Winter Blues: Seasonal Affective Disorder* (New York: Guilford Press, 1993).

Chapter 16

Beaulieu, John. *Music and Sound in the Healing Arts* (New York: Station Hill Press, 1987).

Narby, Jeremy, and Francis Huxley, eds. *Shamans Through Time: 500 Years on the Path to Knowledge* (New York: Putnam Publishing Group, 2001).

Steiger, Brad. *Totems: The Transformative Power of Your Personal Animal Totem* (San Francisco: HarperSanFrancisco, 1997).

Chapter 17

Buckland, Raymond. *Practical Candleburning Rituals* (St. Paul: Llewellyn Publications, 1985).

Kavasch, E. Barrie, and Karen Baar. *American Indian Healing Arts: Herbs, Rituals, and Remedies for Every Season of Life* (New York: Bantam Books, 1999)

Tisserand, Robert. *The Art of Aromatherapy* (Rochester, VT: Inner Traditions International, 1978).

Chapter 18

Paterson, Helena. *The Celtic Lunar Zodiac* (St. Paul: Llewellyn Publications, 2001).

Seymour, Percy. *The Scientific Basis of Astrology: Tuning to the Music of the Planets* (New York: St. Martin's Press, 1992).

Chapter 19

Jackson, Phil. *Sacred Hoops* (New York: Hyperion, 1995).

Jeitner-Hartmann, Bertrun, and Thomas Thiemeyer. *Magical Labyrinths: Journeys Through Space and Time with Poster* (Kansas City, MO: Andrews & McMeel, 2001).

Johnson-Bennett, Pam. *Think Like a Cat: How to Raise a Well-Adjusted Cat—Not a Sour-Puss* (New York: Penguin USA, 2000).

Reynolds, Rita M. *Blessing the Bridge: What Animals Teach Us about Death, Dying, and Beyond* (Troutdale, OR: NewSage Press, 2000).

Tucker, Toni. *Zen Dog* (New York: Clarkson Potter, 2001).

Chapter 20

Goldstein, Joseph. *Seeking the Heart of Wisdom: The Path of Insight Meditation* (Boston: Shambhala Publications, 2001).

Kabat-Zinn, Jon. *Guided Body Scan* (Worcester: University of Massachusetts Medical Center, 1984).

Khalsa, Dharma Singh, and Cameron Stauth. *Meditation as Medicine* (New York: Pocket Books, 2001).

Kornfield, Jack. *After the Ecstasy, the Laundry: How the Heart Grows Wise on the Spiritual Path* (New York: Bantam Books, 2001).

Chapter 21

Adapted from Lopez, Donald S., Jr. *Prisoners of Shangri-La.* (University of Chicago Press: 1998; pps. 182–3).

Orenstein, Robert. *The Right Mind: Making Sense of the Hemispheres* (New York: Harcourt Brace & Co., 1997).

Schwartz, Mark. S. *Biofeedback: A Practitioner's Guide* (New York: Guilford Press, 1995).

Walker, Evan Harris. *The Physics of Consciousness: The Quantum Minds and the Meaning of Life* (Cambridge, MA: Perseus Books Group, 2001).

Selected Medical
Articles and Links

Frecsa E. Neuro-ontological Interpretation of Spiritual Experiences. *Neuropsychophamacol Hung.* 2006 Oct; 8 (3): 143–53.

Habler HJ. Coordination of Sympathetic and Respiratory Systems: Neurophysiological Experiments. *Clin Exp Hypertension.* 1995 Jan–Feb; 17 (1–2): 223–35.

Jella SA. The Effects of Unilateral Forced Nostril Breathing on Cognitive Performance. *IntJ Neuroscie.* 1993 Nov; 73 (1–2): 61–8.

Jerath, R., J. W. Edry, V. A. Barnes and V. Jerath (2006). Physiology of Long Pranayamic Breathing: Neural Respiratory Elements May Provide a Mechanism that Explains How Slow Deep Breathing Shifts the Autonomic Nervous System. *Med Hypotheses* 67 (3): 566–71.

Kozhevnikov M. The Enhancement of Visuospatial Processing Efficiency Through Buddhist Deity Meditation. *Psychol Sci.* 2009 May; 20 (5): 645–53.

Mayo Clinic on Meditation. Website: *www.mayoclinic.com/health/meditation/HQ01070*

Morone NE. "I Felt Like a New Person." The Effects of Mindfulness Meditation on Older Adults with Chronic Pain: Qualitative Narrative Analysis of Daily Diary Entries. *L Pain.* 2008 Sep; 9 (9): 841–8. Epub 2008 Jun 12.

National Center for Complementary and Alternative Medicine (NCCAM), a division of the National Institutes of Health (NIH). Meditation website: *http://nccam.nih.gov/health/meditation*

Pilowsky P. Good Vibrations? Respiratory Rhythms in Central Control of Blood Pressure. *Clin Exp Pharmcol Physiol.* 1995 Sept; 22 (9): 594–604.

Pramanik T. Immediate Effect of Slow Pace Bhastika Pranayama on Blood Pressure and Heart Rate. *J Altern Complement medi.* 2009 Mar; 15 (3): 293–5.

Sequeira H. Electrical Autonomic Correlates of Emotion. *J Psychophysiol.* 2009 Jan; 71(1): 50–6.

Vera FM. Subjective Sleep Quality and Hormonal Modulation in Long-Term Yoga Practitioners. *Biol Pschol.* 2009 Jul; 8 (3): 164–8.

Wu SD. Inward-Attention Meditation Increases Parasympathetic Activity: A Study Based on Heart Rate Variability. *Biomed Res.* 2008 Oct; 29 (5): 245–50.

CD Contents

Track 1: Standard Twice Daily Practice (Morning and Evening) 15:02

Track 2: The Three Assignments 1:36

Track 3: Five Minute Mid-Day Refresh 4:50

Track 4: Embryonic Breathing 1:50

Track 5: Lakshmi Mantra 17:55

Track 6: Peace Meditation 0:53

Track 7: A Prayer for Lovingkindness 2:19

Track 8: The Still, Small Voice (based on 1 Kings 19:11–13) 2:02

Track 9: From *Saint Patrick's Breastplate* 2:59

Track 10: From the *Canticle to the Sun* 1:46

Track 11: A Meditation of Hildegard of Bingen 1:23

Track 12: A Rumi Poem: One Whisper of the Beloved 1:50

Track 13: A Sikh Meditation 1:12

Track 14: From Patanjali's *Yoga Sutras* 4:11

Track 15: Mahatma Gandhi: Thoughts on Self-Transformation and World Transformation 2:13

Index

CD Credits

The Three Assignments [0:01:33]
Waves on Beach from Freesound by Acclivity

Twenty Minute Breath Control and Energy Work
[0:18:55]
Pensive Vibes 3–5 by Daniel Cantor © 2010

Five Minute Mid-Day Refresh [0:04:48]
Magic Gong from Freesound by Gezortenplotz

Aum Sharavanabhava [0:10:58]
Misra Shivranjani Tanpura by Gretchen Ruckert ©
2009 at Notable.com

Great Compassion Mantra [0:10:06]
Tibetan Chant from Freesound by DJ Griffin

Great Compassion Mantra [0:10:06]
Excerpt from "Heart Sutra" sung by Geshe Gendun
from *Many Paths, One Joy* by Robert Jonas © 2005
at Notable.com. Courtesy of Emptybell.org

From Patanjali's Yoga Sutras [0:04:09]
Desh performed by George Ruckert © 2009 at
Notable.com

Peace Meditation [0:00:50]
Tibetan Chant from Freesound by DJ Griffin

A Sikh Meditation [0:01:10]
Pensive Vibes 6&7 by Daniel Cantor © 2010

A Prayer for Lovingkindness [0:02:17]
Birds from Freesound by Crk365

The Still, Small Voice (based on 1 Kings 19:11–13)
[0:02:00]
Flute played by Nathan Berla-Shulock © 2010

Embryonic Breathing [0:01:48]
Gongs by Daniel Cantor © 2010

From the Canticle of the Sun [0:01:54]
Excerpt from "O Virtus Sapentia" sung by June
Boyce-Tillman from *Many Paths, One Joy* by Robert Jonas © 2005 at Notable.com. Courtesy of
Emptybell.org

A Meditation of Hildegard of Bingen [0:01:21]
Catherine Meyer, Pipe Organist, performing *Dietrich Buxtehude: Praeludium in G*, BuxWV 149 live
at Marsh Chapel. Recorded by Notable.com C.
Meyer © 2005

A Rumi Poem: One Whisper of the Beloved
[0:01:48]
Dumbek and Finger Cymbals by Daniel Cantor
© 2010

Mahatma Ghandi: Thoughts on Self-Transformation
and World Transformation [0:02:13]
Digital Tanpura by Daniel Cantor © 2010